Fluid Therapy
for Veterinary Technicians and Nurses

Fluid Therapy
for Veterinary Technicians and Nurses

Charlotte Donohoe, RVT, VTS (ECC)

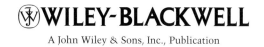

WILEY-BLACKWELL

A John Wiley & Sons, Inc., Publication

Registered office: John Wiley & Sons Ltd, The Atrium, Southern Gate, Chichester, West Sussex, PO19 8SQ, UK

Editorial offices: 2121 State Avenue, Ames, Iowa 50014-8300, USA
  The Atrium, Southern Gate, Chichester, West Sussex, PO19 8SQ, UK
  9600 Garsington Road, Oxford, OX4 2DQ, UK

For details of our global editorial offices, for customer services and for information about how to apply for permission to reuse the copyright material in this book please see our website at www.wiley.com/wiley-blackwell.

Library of Congress Cataloging-in-Publication Data

Donohoe, Charlotte.
  Fluid therapy for veterinary technicians and nurses / Charlotte Donohoe.
      p. ; cm.
  Includes bibliographical references and index.
  ISBN 978-0-8138-1484-1 (pbk. : alk. paper)
  I. Title.
  [DNLM: 1. Fluid Therapy–veterinary. 2. Body Fluids–physiology. 3. Veterinary Medicine–methods.
4. Water-Electrolyte Imbalance–veterinary. SF 910.W38]
  636.089'63992–dc23
                            2011036435

A catalogue record for this book is available from the British Library.

Wiley also publishes its books in a variety of electronic formats. Some content that appears in print may not be available in electronic books.

Set in 10/12 pt Sabon by Toppan Best-set Premedia Limited
Printed and bound in Singapore by Markono Print Media Pte Ltd

1 2012

To my parents: Thank you for always believing in me and for constantly supporting me, no matter what the endeavor.

To my husband and my children: Thank you for your patience, your understanding, and your love, help, and support through this enormous project. I couldn't have done this without you.

To my mentor, Dr. Karol Mathews: You are a special human being. I hope you realize the impact that you have had throughout your career. You inspired me, you encouraged me, and you believed in me. Thank you so much for giving me the opportunity to explore the limits of my capabilities. It has been quite an adventure.

Contents

PowerPoint documents of figures and PDFs of questions and answers available for download at www.wiley.com/go/donohoenursing.

Preface

As the practices of veterinary nursing and veterinary technology evolve, technicians are blessed with more and more responsibility. As our profession grows, we must accept new challenges and strive to maintain a level of knowledge and technical skills that allows us to perform routine as well as unexpected procedures with grace and confidence.

Fluid therapy is fundamental to many aspects of small animal practice. Its role is multifaceted because fluids are used as a supportive measure in surgical patients, as a means of nutrition in hospitalized patients, and as the backbone of therapy in severely compromised animals.

Given that the role of fluid therapy is so important, the objective of the technician should be fluency in all of its aspects. The technician is responsible for obtaining and maintaining intravenous access, monitoring a patient's responses to fluid therapy, and noticing and reacting appropriately to unexpected or undesired changes in a patient's condition that are a result of therapeutic interventions.

To carry out these responsibilities, we must be well versed in the principles that guide fluid therapy. There are many opportunities for technicians to further their education with respect to fluid therapy. However, these are often either too basic or too advanced with respect to the information covered. This text has been compiled with the goal of bridging the gap between these two extremes.

Small animal practices often rely on their technicians to provide current, safe, and practical technical expertise with respect to catheter placement and monitoring of intravenous fluid therapy. This text includes details related to these areas that can help guide technicians in deciding the appropriate approach to intravenous therapy for their respective practice.

In addition, information pertaining to long-term fluid therapy, intravenous nutrition, varieties of equipment, and potential complications associated with fluid therapy has also been included.

This text presents technician students with a wealth of new information with which they can put new skills and ideas to safe use. It offers experienced technicians new ideas, additional information, and detailed facts to support their current role while increasing their knowledge base. For advanced care technicians, this text solidifies the rationale behind many of the techniques and theories learned on the job while presenting new information and differing opinions for consideration.

Acknowledgments

All of the illustrations in this text were created by Rachel Wallach. Rachel, I can't thank you enough for sharing your time, your creativity, and your generosity with me throughout this project.

I would like to include a special thank you to Vicki Titus and Holly for their patience, their eagerness to help, and their special contribution to the cover of this book.

Charlotte Donohoe

Fluid Therapy
for Veterinary Technicians and Nurses

Body Water

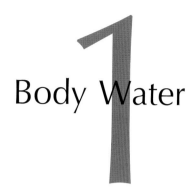

Body water is typically described by referring to how much of an animal's body weight it represents. It is most often defined as a percentage and thus can be calculated for any patient. In the average healthy animal, total body water is equivalent to 60% of total body weight. An animal's body condition must be considered before determining the expected volume of body water. Because fat contains little or no water, an obese animal will have less than 60% of its body weight devoted to water. Animals that are excessively thin have a higher percentage of weight, roughly 70% as body water. Neonates also differ from the average healthy adult because water comprises roughly 80% of their body weight (Michell et al., 1989).

Body water is housed in several different compartments. Of the 60% of body weight that is fluid, 40% is maintained in the intracellular fluid space (ICF) and 20% in the extracellular fluid space (ECF) (Wellman et al., 2006). Although the extracellular space houses a smaller volume of body water than the intracellular space, it is an extremely important consideration during fluid therapy.

In illness, fluid loss occurs through different routes. Initial losses may cause a disturbance in one of the body's compartments, but these losses eventually are distributed and shared across all compartments (Fig. 1.1A, B). Water is borrowed from one space to replenish another. The compartments that are smallest by comparison experience a more significant impact from their loss than the larger compartments. Because the extracellular space is small to begin with, losses from this space must be addressed, and it is the first compartment that is replenished by intravenous fluid therapy.

Much of the extracellular fluid is found in the tissues, bathing the cells, and is referred to as interstitial fluid (ISF). This ISF represents approximately three-quarters of the total ECF, translating into about 15% of the patient's body weight. The remainder of the ECF is found in the vascular space and represents 5% of total body weight. Body water housed

Fluid Therapy for Veterinary Technicians and Nurses, First Edition. Charlotte Donohoe.
© 2012 Charlotte Donohoe. Published 2012 by John Wiley & Sons, Inc.

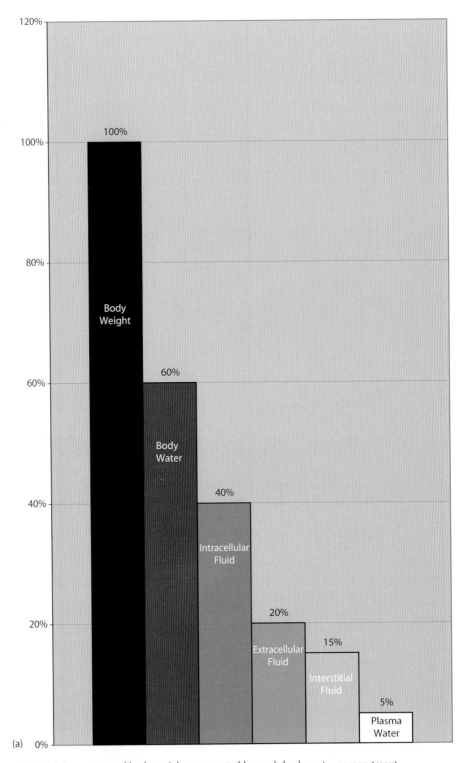

Figure 1.1. (a) Percentages of body weight represented by each body water compartment.

Body Water Compartments

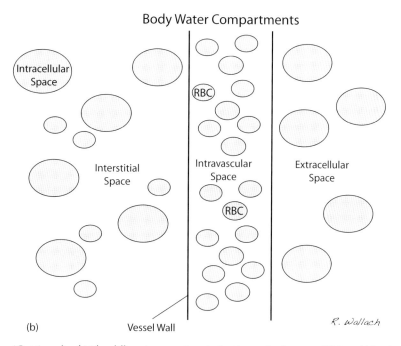

Figure 1.1. (*Continued*) (b) The different compartments that house body water. RBC, red blood cells. Illustration by Rachel Wallach.

within the vasculature is referred to as plasma, the noncellular portion of the blood. At first glance it may seem that these numbers do not play a vital role in the day-to-day routine of the veterinary technician. However, it is important to recognize that without the ability to estimate the fluid volume in the extracellular compartment, we cannot plan appropriate fluid therapy to support or replenish our compromised patients.

The synovial joints, the aqueous chambers of the eyes, and the cerebrospinal space contain a small portion of ECF (~1% body weight) and are known as the transcellular fluid compartments (Wellman 2006) (Fig. 1.2).

In the healthy animal the movement of fluid throughout these compartments is well controlled. There is a natural tendency for water to move in a manner that will balance the solute concentrations between compartments. Solutes are the dissolved substances that reside within body fluids. When the solute concentration of a compartment is altered, water moves into the compartment with the higher solute concentration to restore balance.

Body water compartments are separated by a semipermeable membrane, which means that water and certain solutes may pass through the membrane and others may not. The process of **osmosis** occurs when water passes through a semipermeable membrane and is drawn toward a space that has a higher solute concentration (Wellman 2006). Movement of water into an area of higher solute concentration dilutes the solute and reinstates equilibrium.

For the various body water compartments to carry out their physiologic responsibilities, it is sometimes necessary to maintain water within a compartment and prevent its movement into higher solute areas. Various solutes within the compartments are responsible for this regulation. Due to their inability to pass freely through semipermeable membranes, these solutes exert a force on the interior of their respective compartment.

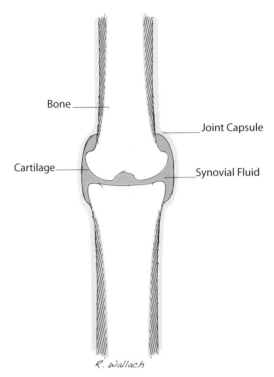

Figure 1.2. The synovial joint is one of the potential spaces that houses a small portion of the extracellular body water. Illustration by Rachel Wallach.

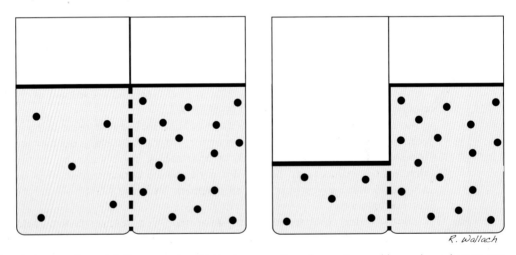

Figure 1.3. Osmosis is the process by which water moves through a semipermeable membrane from an area of lower solute concentration to an area of higher solute concentration. The result is that the solute concentration on either side of the membrane is the same. Illustration by Rachel Wallach.

This force, referred to as *osmotic pressure,* is the amount of force required to keep water within a compartment (Guyton and Hall 2000d). A compartment with higher solute concentration has greater osmotic pressure. This compartment exerts the stronger pull (between two compartments) and draws water toward it, across the semipermeable membrane (Fig. 1.3).

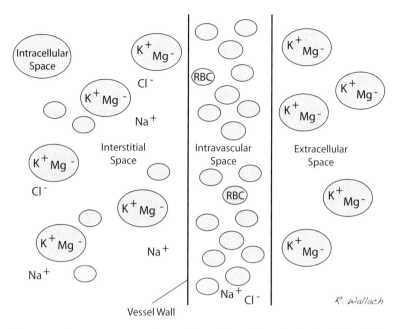

Figure 1.4. The appropriate compartments for a variety of ions. Illustration by Rachel Wallach.

Electrolytes and their fluid compartments

The extracellular and intracellular fluid compartments contain different concentrations of important solutes called ions, which are electrically charged particles found throughout the body water compartments. The term *electrolyte* refers to the combination of ions to form a substance that will break down in water.

Electrolytes have an important role in maintaining acid-base status within the body. A second but no less important role of electrolytes is to provide osmotic pressure and regulate the movement of body water between compartments.

The extracellular and intracellular spaces contain high concentrations of sodium (Na^+) and chloride (Cl^-) and potassium (K^+) and magnesium (Mg^{++}), respectively (Guyton and Hall 2000c) (Fig. 1.4).

Sodium has a positive electrical charge associated with it and referred to as a cation. It is the most plentiful cation in the ECF. Sodium plays an important role in maintaining the volume of water in the extracellular compartment. It is exchanged between the intracellular and extracellular compartments with ease. Each cell membrane houses a pump that exchanges sodium for potassium. When sodium concentration reaches an unsuitable level within the cell, the sodium potassium pump removes a sodium ion (positive charge) in exchange for a potassium ion (positive charge) (Wellman et al., 2006) (Fig. 1.5). This mechanism maintains a higher concentration of sodium outside the cell, making it an important regulator of osmosis (water will diffuse into areas of higher sodium concentration).

Chloride has a negative charge associated with it and is referred to as an anion. It is the most abundant anion in the ECF compartment. It too can move in and out of cells. The ECF also contains a substantial amount of bicarbonate and a small amount of

Na$^+$/K$^+$ Pump

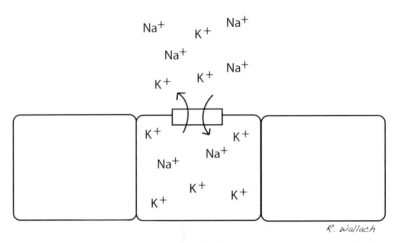

Figure 1.5. The sodium potassium pump is responsible for moderating the exchange of sodium and potassium between the intracellular and extracellular spaces. Illustration by Rachel Wallach.

potassium. Despite their smaller numbers, these ions have important physiologic roles and impart severe consequences when their concentrations are altered.

The ICF compartment is characterized by high concentrations of potassium (cation) and magnesium (anion). Potassium is vital to normal cellular metabolism due to its important influence has on the movement of water into and out of the cell. Disease(s) causing damage to, or death of, cells results in cellular potassium leaking into the extracellular space. This is of particular interest in the clinical setting when we consider how often we see abnormalities in serum potassium levels. Hyperkalemia, the condition in which the level of potassium within the blood is elevated, can lead to severe arrhythmias (Stepien 1999). In particular, bradyarrhythmias and cardiac arrest are significant concerns with hyperkalemic patients. Magnesium, phosphate, and protein molecules also impart a regulatory influence on the movement of water between compartments.

The concentration of electrolytes within a solution can be expressed in several different ways. One of the formats encountered frequently in fluid therapy is millimoles per liter (mmol/L). This measurement denotes the molecular weight of the electrolyte in a volume of solvent (Wellman 2006).

Water Gain and Water Loss

The volume of water that normally exists in the body is fairly consistent. Animals have two primary means of obtaining water: drinking and eating. A normal healthy animal regulates its drinking based on its body's requirements. For example, the body of an animal that has been exposed to an extremely hot environment is likely to lose a larger volume of body water than normal due to its panting (increased loss of water via respiratory tract) than an animal resting in a cool indoor environment. The loss of water from the ECF compartment lowers the concentration of water and increases solute concentrations in that compartment. This decrease in water concentration in the ECF compartment sets in motion a chain of activities, ultimately resulting in an increased water demand (increased thirst).

In the literature, a wide range of values is published for the volume of water normally consumed by a healthy animal in one day. In canines, water consumption varies between 50 and 100 mL/kg per day, whereas felines are expected to consume somewhere between 40 and 70 mL/kg per day (Wellman 2006). The volume of water obtained through an animal's diet can vary depending on the type of food consumed. Canned food has a higher water content than dry kibble, and as a result, animals on a canned diet consume less water than those on a dry diet. Semi-moist kibble is also available for canines and felines. This type of diet falls in the middle of the moisture range, containing more water than kibble but less than canned food.

Dietary proteins, carbohydrates, and fats are broken down into smaller blocks as they are digested. Carbohydrates are reduced into simple sugars, fats into fatty acids and glycerol, and protein into amino acids. One of the processes involved in digestion is oxidation, defined as the combination of a substance with oxygen. Water is one of the products of this process and as such is made available to the body through the digestion of food (Guyton and Hall 2000a). Regardless of the type of diet, the metabolism of it produces small amounts of water.

Water is removed from the body in three ways. It is excreted in the urine, excreted in the stool, and lost via the skin and respiratory tract. The body ultimately attempts to maintain balance between compartments despite continuous gains and losses of body water. Fluid must be exchanged between compartments to maintain this balance. Osmosis is the primary process through which water is exchanged between compartments. Several circumstances influence when water is exchanged between compartments. As previously discussed, solute concentration regulates movement of water across a semipermeable membrane. The use of fluid therapy involves many different solutes that are most often delivered into the intravascular space. In light of their contribution to fluid therapy, we discuss plasma proteins and sodium and chloride, the solutes, and the roles they play in the movement of fluid between compartments.

Plasma protein

The protein molecules found within the plasma are large in size and have a high molecular weight. In solution, particles with a high molecular weight are called colloids. An important characteristic of plasma proteins is their contribution to osmotic pressure. When referring specifically to the force exerted by plasma proteins, it is acceptable to use the terms *oncotic pressure* and *colloid osmotic pressure* interchangeably (Wellman 2006).

Recall from the discussion regarding osmotic pressure that solutes that cannot pass through a semipermeable membrane exert force on one side of the membrane and draw water into their compartment. The same is true of proteins. Protein molecules are large and do not readily fit through most capillary pores. In health, the concentration of plasma proteins in the vascular compartment is higher than that throughout the interstitium (Guyton and Hall 2000b).

Colloidal osmotic pressure is one of the important forces governing the movement of fluids throughout the extracellular compartment (between the interstitium and intravascular spaces). This is of particular interest in two situations frequently encountered in fluid therapy.

Hypovolemic shock is a condition encountered in veterinary patients and with frequency in emergency medicine. It arises from a depletion of intravascular volume that is typically precipitated by trauma, severe acute disease, or prolonged illness (Wingfield 2002). Patients that suffer from hypovolemic shock experience a subsequent decrease in cardiac output and blood pressure (hypotension). Blood flow is prioritized to areas that are vital to the animal's survival. Blood flow to the periphery is diminished. Tissue perfusion (flow of blood) in these areas is maintained or minimized, respectively.

Hypovolemic patients require administration of fluid therapy to preserve perfusion to vital organs; this is accomplished by increasing the intravascular volume. In severe cases of cardiovascular collapse, fluids known as colloids are occasionally used as a component of therapy. *Colloids* are fluids rich in large molecules and as such tend to stay in the vascular space (they are too large to pass through healthy capillaries). They add to the colloid osmotic pressure within the vascular space, which encourages fluid from the extravascular space to shift into the vasculature. The increase in vascular volume means an increase in venous return and consequently an increase in CO.

In patients suspected of having damaged or leaky capillaries, plasma proteins become an important consideration for a different reason than increasing colloid osmotic pressure. Where they can be used to a patient's benefit in the previous example, the use of colloids can be detrimental in disease states that alter capillary permeability, such as in cases of sepsis or with burn victims (Dhupa 2002). Leaky capillaries cannot effectively maintain large molecules within the intravascular space. If proteins escape into the interstitium, body water will follow. This movement of body water will upset the balance between compartments and lead to interstitial edema (Dhupa 2002). Colloids (synthetic or natural) must be avoided or be used with extreme caution in patients experiencing disease or injury that compromises the integrity of the capillaries.

Solutes and their influence

Solute molecules, such as sodium and chloride, move between the vascular and interstitial spaces with greater ease than protein molecules. However, this does not preclude these ions from having an extreme influence on the movement of body water (Fig. 1.6).

Fluids developed for use in medical settings have varying amounts of solute concentrations providing flexibility to tailor the fluid therapy to specific patient needs. It is helpful, then, to understand how the delivery of hypertonic, hypotonic, and isotonic solutions to the intravascular compartment affects therapy.

A fluid is considered *isotonic* if it has the same solute concentration as the one to which it is being compared. Of particular interest to veterinary technicians is the comparison with the ECF. If an isotonic solution is delivered intravenously, it will distribute evenly throughout the interstitial and intravascular spaces. Because there are no dramatic differences in solute concentration, there is no significant shift of water between compartments. The delivery of an isotonic fluid increases the volume of the entire extracellular compartment. Normal saline (0.9% NaCl) is an example of an isotonic fluid.

A *hypotonic* fluid has a solute concentration lower than that of the ECF. When delivered intravascularly, this fluid causes a shift of water into the cellular space so that the solute concentration of extracellular fluid returns to normal. Both compartments (ICF

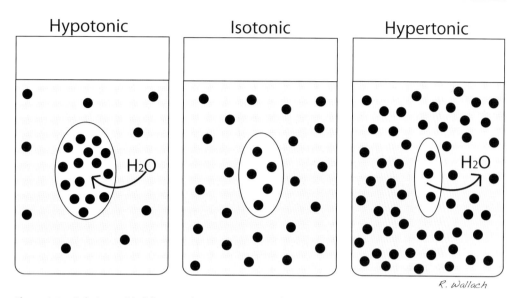

Figure 1.6. Solutions with different solute concentrations have specific effects on the cell. Isotonic solutions do not cause extensive movement of water (H_2O) into or out of the cell. Hypertonic solutions cause movement of H_2O out of the cell. Hypotonic solutions cause movement of H_2O into the cell. Illustration by Rachel Wallach.

and ECF) end up with an overall increase in volume, but the gain is more substantial within the cells. An example of a hypotonic solution is 0.45% sodium chloride.

Hypertonic fluids have a higher solute concentration than that of the ECF. Addition of this fluid to the intravascular space causes a dramatic increase in solute concentration, causing water to move from the interstitium and the intracellular space into the vasculature. This large movement of water then dilutes the solute concentration to return the vascular compartment to its normal solute concentration. An example of a hypertonic solution is 7% sodium chloride.

Hypertonic fluids must be used with caution because they borrow water from the intracellular compartment. Dehydrated patients have little to spare in their intracellular compartment, and adjunctive therapy is often needed to protect these cells from further fluid loss.

Chapter Summary

Body water represents 60% of body weight in the healthy animal. The volume of water housed within the body is divided into different compartments called the intracellular and extracellular spaces. The intracellular space identifies all that water housed within the cells throughout the body. The extracellular space contains the remainder of body water that is found outside of the cells. The extracellular space is further divided into the intravascular and interstitial spaces. The interstitial compartment holds water found between the cells but not within the vasculature. The intravascular space corresponds to the water that circulates throughout the vasculature at any given time. The body water within the vascular space is the noncellular component of blood and is also referred to as plasma.

Electrolytes are combinations of ions that break down in water. Their balance is of critical importance to the health of all animals. Different electrolytes are found in specific concentrations in the intracellular and extracellular compartments.

Colloid osmotic pressure, or oncotic pressure, refers to the strong force exerted by proteins found in plasma. These proteins are too large to pass through semipermeable membranes. They exert a force across the membrane that helps maintain the balance of water in its respective compartment.

Fluids that influence flow of water into and out of the cellular space can be isotonic, hypotonic, or hypertonic. Isotonic fluids have the same solute concentration as the intracellular space. Hypotonic fluids have a lower solute concentration than the intracellular space. Hypertonic fluids have a higher solute concentration than the intracellular space. These cause no net change in movement of water, a net movement of water into the cell, and a net movement of water out of the cell, respectively.

Review Questions

1. What percentage of body weight is composed of water in the average healthy animal?
2. Is the percentage of body weight represented by water higher or lower in neonates than in adults?
3. The water housed within the intravascular space contributes approximately what percentage of body weight?
4. What is osmosis?
5. What are the two main electrolytes found in the extracellular space?
6. Which electrolytes are found primarily in the intracellular space?
7. Which molecules contribute to oncotic pressure within the vasculature?
8. Fill in the blanks with the correct answer.
   Hypovolemic shock is a condition in which patients experience a decrease in
   _____ and _____ due to a loss of volume from their intravascular space.
   a. Packed cell volume and blood pressure
   b. Cardiac output and heart rate
   c. Packed cell volume and heart rate
   d. Cardiac output and blood pressure

Answers to the review questions can be found on page 221 in the Appendix. The review questions are also available for download on a companion website at www.wiley.com/go/donohoenursing.

Further Reading

Dhupa, N. 2002. Burn injury. In W. Wingfield and M. Raffe M., eds. *The Veterinary ICU Book*, 973–981. Jackson, WY: Teton NewMedia.

Guyton, A., and J. Hall. 2000a. Dietary balances; regulation of feeding; obesity and starvation; vitamins and minerals. In *Textbook of Medical Physiology*, 803–814. Philadelphia: Saunders.

Guyton, A., and J. Hall. 2000b. The microcirculation and the lymphatic system: capillary fluid exchange, interstitial fluid, and lymph flow. In *Textbook of Medical Physiology*, 162–174. Philadelphia: Saunders.

Guyton, A., and J. Hall. 2000c. The body fluid compartments: extracellular and intracellular fluids; interstitial fluid and edema. In *Textbook of Medical Physiology*, 264–278. Philadelphia: Saunders.

Guyton, A., and J. Hall. 2000d. Transport of substances through the cell membrane. In *Textbook of Medical Physiology*, 40–51. Philadelphia: Saunders.

Michell, A., R. Bywater, et al. 1989. Regulation of body fluids. In *Veterinary Fluid Therapy*, 1–19. Oxford, UK: Blackwell.

Stepien, R. 1999. Cardiovascular emergencies. In *Manual of Canine and Feline Emergency and Critical Care*, 37–63. Cheltenham, UK: BSAVA.

Wellman, M., S. DiBartola, and C. Kohn. 2006. Applied physiology of body fluids in dogs and cats. In DiBartola, S., ed. *Fluid, Electrolyte, and Acid-Base Disorders in Small Animal Practice*, 3–25. St. Louis: Saunders.

Wingfield, W.E. 2002. Fluid and electrolyte therapy. In W.E. Wingfield and M. R. Raffe, eds. *The Veterinary ICU Book*, 167–188. Jackson, WY: Teton NewMedia.

Patient Assessment 2

In many cases the veterinary technician is the first person to evaluate a patient presenting to the clinic with some degree of urgency. A brief examination can gather pertinent information with respect to the hydration and volume status of the patient. Note that hydration (normal or dehydrated) and volume status (normo/hypovolemia) are not synonymous. They are often seen together but can also be present alone, and each should be evaluated in every patient.

Dehydration

The terms *dehydration* and *hypovolemia* are often used interchangeably; however, it is incorrect to do so. Each term refers to a separate condition affecting the body. Hypovolemia and dehydration are often concurrent in emergency patients but can occur independently as well.

Dehydration is a condition that arises when excessive amounts of body water are lost. This deficit causes water from within the cells to move into the extracellular space. Some of this water also redistributes to the vasculature (Mensack 2008). Hypovolemia refers to a deficit in fluid volume that is circulating throughout the body. The intravascular space is the compartment most affected by hypovolemia, and as such, initial therapy for this condition can differ from the treatment of dehydration.

Fluid Therapy for Veterinary Technicians and Nurses, First Edition. Charlotte Donohoe.
© 2012 Charlotte Donohoe. Published 2012 by John Wiley & Sons, Inc.

Dehydration

The extravascular compartment includes the cells and the space surrounding the cells (interstitium). Each cell is responsible for a specific function and requires specific conditions to fulfill these responsibilities. The interstitial compartment must provide an environment that is suitable for the cells to thrive. In other words, the compartment must house a liquid medium via which nutrition can be supplied to the cells. To meet these requirements, a fine balance of fluid is maintained.

Conditions may arise causing a disruption of the fluid balance in these compartments. As previously mentioned, dehydration is caused by excessive loss of water from the body. Types of dehydration can be described in relation to the amount of other solutes that remain in the compartments.

Hypotonic dehydration describes loss of water that has a low concentration of dissolved particles. Patients with chronic congestive heart failure eventually develop this type of dehydration if left untreated. The solute concentration within the compartment is greater than that of the fluid lost.

Hypertonic dehydration involves the loss of fluid that has a high solute concentration. This type of dehydration can be caused by exercise, anxiety-producing events, or even heat stroke (DiBartola and Bateman 2006).

Isotonic dehydration is caused by many disease processes. Vomiting, anorexia, diarrhea, and hemorrhagic shock are common causes of isotonic dehydration. Body water that is lost has a solute concentration equal to that which remains in the compartment.

Hypovolemia

Hypovolemia is the condition in which there is a decrease in the volume of blood circulating within the vasculature. The vascular space contains blood (the cellular portion of intravascular body water) and blood plasma (the noncellular portion). Hypovolemia refers to the loss of blood plasma and/or blood from the intravascular space.

Blood plasma is composed of approximately 90% water and carries dissolved proteins, glucose, and carbon dioxide. It is where the blood cells are suspended and the means by which they are transported throughout the vasculature.

The vascular system transports blood and blood plasma throughout the entire body. It carries oxygenated blood to the tissues and carries carbon dioxide and other waste products away from the tissues back to the organs for processing. This system relies heavily on the heart for its ability to contract and send newly oxygenated blood back into systemic circulation. Organs and tissues depend on the circulating blood volume and suffer varying degrees of damage when that volume is not delivered, as is found in hypovolemic states.

In sickness, intravascular volume can be depleted in a variety of ways, ultimately leading to hypovolemia if the disease process is left untreated. Trauma, toxin ingestion, prolonged vomiting or diarrhea, severe hemorrhage, and conditions causing extreme vasodilation (sepsis, anaphylaxis) are common causes of hypovolemia.

Fluid loss that involves a higher proportion of solute than water causes movement of water from the extracellular space toward the intracellular compartment. Some of this water is borrowed from the intravascular space (Mensack 2008). The loss of fluid volume from the intravascular space leads to hypovolemia if the condition causing the fluid loss is left untreated.

Animals that experience massive hemorrhage also enter a hypovolemic state as their intravascular volume is depleted through direct loss of blood from one or more vessels.

Evaluating Patient Hydration and Volume Status

Clinical evaluation of hydration status begins with the physical examination. The veterinary technician should begin the assessment of the patient with an initial hands-off visual assessment of the animal's overall demeanor. A patient's critical illness (or lack thereof) cannot be diagnosed solely based on their demeanor; however, it is an important observation to make and include in the overall assessment. The animal's attitude may indicate how significantly it is affected by its current volume and hydration status.

An entire thorough physical examination may not frequently be performed by the technician, but a preliminary evaluation is warranted in any patient that presents to the hospital with even the slightest of health concerns. The technician can initiate the assessment of the patient's hydration status by measuring the following parameters.

Skin turgor/skin tent

Skin turgor refers to the elasticity of an animal's skin. It is evaluated by measuring the skin's ability to return to its normal shape and position. *Skin tent* is the term used to describe not only the process by which turgor is evaluated but also the shape that the skin is stretched into to observe its elasticity. Several areas on the patient's body can be used to evaluate a skin tent. The most frequently used area is the skin on the dorsal aspect of the neck slightly cranial to the scapulae. Additional sites for skin tent evaluation include the skin over the thoracic vertebrae, over one scapula, along the dorsum, or on the dorsal aspect of the skull between the ears. It is advisable to tent the patient's skin in more than one location to fully evaluate the skin turgor (Figs. 2.1 and 2.2).

In a normal, adequately hydrated patient, a skin tent typically returns to its normal position within 1 to 2 seconds. The technician may notice a slight delay in skin repositioning in a patient that is approaching 5%–6% dehydration. An increase in the duration of the skin tent is definitely noticeable by 6%–8% dehydration, and a patient whose skin remains in a tented shape is likely approaching the 10%–12% dehydration range (Miller et al., 1992).

 Nursing considerations

Note the age and body weight of each patient when evaluating skin tent/turgor. Geriatric and overly lean patients may have a prolonged skin tent, whereas juvenile or obese patients may maintain skin elasticity (have normal skin tent) despite dehydration.

It is important to remember that this is a subjective test that cannot be used alone to determine an estimation of hydration status. It should be used along with other information garnered throughout the physical examination to provide a reasonable estimate of patient hydration.

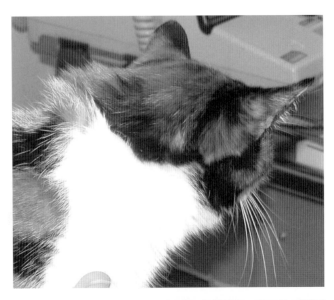

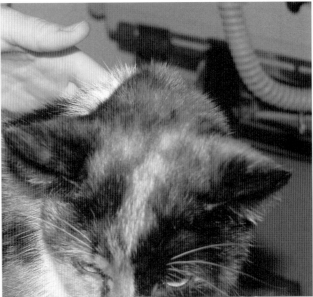

Figures 2.1 and 2.2. Skin tent. The skin is raised and observed as it returns to normal. A prolonged skin tent can be a sign of dehydration.

Mucous membrane moisture

Every preliminary examination performed by the technician should include the evaluation of mucous membrane (MM) characteristics (Fig. 2.3). With respect to hydration status, MM moisture is of particular interest. MM moisture is most often assessed using a patient's gums. (Although other areas are accessible for evaluation of capillary refill time, they are not quite as helpful as the gums for assessment of MM moisture.) To assess MM moisture in the oral cavity, the lateral aspect of the lip is lifted and gentle

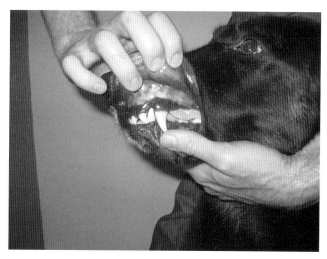

Figure 2.3. Checking mucous membranes. Color and moisture of mucous membranes helps identify dehydration and poor circulation if present.

pressure is applied to the gums just above the gum line. The level of moisture on the buccal side of the lip can also be noted. The technician should note whether the MMs feel moist and slightly slippery (normal), excessively moist and slippery, or dry and slightly tacky/sticky (possible sign of dehydration). Patients often have noticeably dry gums by the time they are estimated at 6%–8% dehydrated. A patient that is 10%–12% dehydrated has dry MMs (Miller et al., 1992).

 ## Nursing considerations

MMs must be evaluated as part of a clinical picture because their characteristics can change based on a number of factors. A patient may present with abnormal MM moisture due to a variety of causes. For example, consider whether the patient has been panting (canine) or open-mouthed breathing (feline) before presentation. In these cases, it is not unreasonable to find tacky MM in the patient during the initial assessment. Patients that are experiencing extreme nausea and/or vomiting may present with excessively moist, slippery MM that could wrongly imply that the patient is well hydrated.

Eye position

Eye position is another parameter that may provide clues to the hydration status of a patient during the technician's initial assessment. As with the parameters previously discussed (skin tent, MM moisture), it is important to recall that this evaluation is subjective and should not be used alone to determine the hydration status of an animal.

In normally hydrated animals it is unusual to see severely sunken eyes or eyes that seem to recess into the bony orbit that surrounds them. Animals that present moderately to severely dehydrated often have appreciable space noticeable rostral to the globe of the eye near the medial canthus. The eyes take on a sunken appearance and, in severe cases, can take on a dull appearance as well (Fig. 2.4).

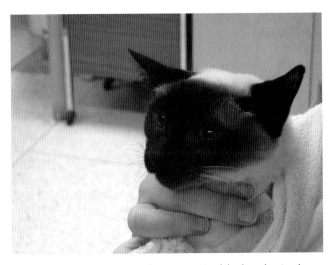

Figure 2.4. Eye position. Sunken eye position is often present in dehydrated animals.

 Nursing considerations

Age, ocular trauma, and retrobulbar and ocular disease can affect the position and appearance of a patient's eyes. Evaluation of eye position and eye clarity is subjective and must be used in conjunction with other physical examination findings to estimate a patient's hydration status.

Mentation

A patient's mentation can vary from one extreme to another depending on the degree of dehydration it is experiencing. It is not difficult to imagine that dehydrated animals will not present as bright and energetic as those with normal hydration and minimal illness. A profoundly dehydrated patient that is also hypovolemic rarely appears bright and alert. The brain is an organ that depends heavily on external sources for energy. It does not maintain its own energy supply. Because its metabolic demands are so high, the brain requires a constant volume of blood circulating to provide sufficient energy to meet its metabolic needs. When these needs are not fully met, the presenting animal may have little energy or interest in his or her surroundings and in extreme cases can be recumbent and stuporous.

 Nursing considerations

Mentation is a characteristic that varies significantly with different types of illness. It is not a parameter that indicates specific degrees of dehydration or hypovolemia but rather is a feature to be noted and considered along with the presenting complaint and initial physical assessment.

Vital parameters

During the initial physical assessment, vital signs can help the technician determine whether a patient's intravascular volume status has been significantly affected by its illness.

In a hypovolemic state, the animal has inadequate blood volume reaching its tissues and organs. The body has compensatory mechanisms to counteract the effects of hypovolemia, but the condition and the process causing it must be reversed to preserve the future health and functionality of the organs.

Heart rate

Cardiac output (CO) is the product of heart rate (HR) and stroke volume (SV) (Miller 2002). SV is the volume of blood pumped into circulation by the left ventricle during one contraction. An increase or decrease in either of these parameters (SV or HR) influences CO in the same direction (a direct relationship). A decrease in the volume of blood circulating within the vasculature results in a smaller volume of blood flowing into the proximal vena cava for delivery to the heart. Decreased blood volume entering the right atrium leads to a decreased SV because less blood returning to the heart supplies less blood to be pumped out of the heart by the left ventricle. The result is that a decrease in circulating blood volume causes a decrease in SV, subsequently decreasing the volume of blood leaving the heart (CO).

Decreased CO causes diminished blood flow to tissues and organs (decreased perfusion). Poor tissue perfusion means that the cells are not receiving adequate oxygen and nutrients for optimal cellular function. Poor perfusion can lead to cell hypoxia and cell death (Wingfield 2002a).

A reduction in circulating blood volume leading to a decrease in systemic blood pressure (BP) is one of the triggers that set in motion a chain of compensatory mechanisms. These mechanisms offer temporary protection for the body's vital organs. The primary goal of these protective measures is to maintain tissue perfusion. These mechanisms provide a degree of protection to vital organs during times of compromised health and poor perfusion (Peitzman 1993).

The chain of events initiated by a decrease in BP is complex and involves many different systems within the body. The following is a condensed version of what transpires.

A decrease in BP is identified by receptors in the major arteries. These receptors are often referred to as baroreceptors or stretch receptors. The following is a very simplified version of the reaction they evoke:

■ Receptors note a fall in BP in one of the main arteries
■ Information is transmitted to brain
■ Brain activates sympathetic nervous system
■ HR and myocardial contractility are increased
■ Vasoconstriction reduces the capacity of the vasculature
■ Venous return increases due to diminished capacity of peripheral vessels

An increase in HR contributes to an increase in CO, which leads to improved perfusion and protects against the effects of hypovolemia. Note that these are temporary short-term measures that the body institutes in the early stages of hypovolemia. Further protective strategies are launched by the body in persistent states of hypovolemia but are beyond the scope of this discussion.

If the veterinary technician's initial assessment of a patient includes a finding of tachycardia, this information should be used in conjunction with the patient's history to begin to assess the patient's volume status.

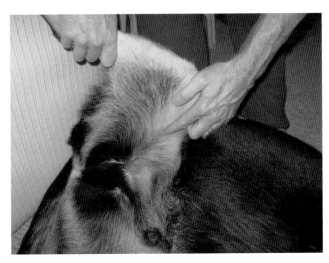

Figure 2.5. The femoral pulse is palpated on the medial aspect of the hind limb. Pulses are evaluated for rate and pulse pressure.

 Nursing consideration

Recall that there are many reasons why a patient's HR may be elevated during the initial examination. Tachycardia is not exclusive to hypovolemia. Pain, anxiety, hypoxia, hyperthermia, and cardiac disease are but a few factors to consider while troubleshooting tachycardia.

Pulse quality

To evaluate the quality of a patient's pulse, the technician should consider how strong the pulse is against the digit, how long it lasts, and whether either of these characteristics fluctuates. Heart rhythm should also be assessed during palpation of pulses and any arrhythmias noted and later recorded via electrocardiogram (ECG).

Pulse pressure should be palpated at a minimum of one site on the patient's body. Ideally, pulses are evaluated in the femoral arteries as well as the dorsal pedal arteries.

Femoral pulses are easily palpated in both feline and canine patients (Fig. 2.5). The pulse is appreciated in the crease between the hind limb and the caudal abdomen at almost the most dorsal point. The artery runs over the femur and can be palpated on the limb side of the crease using very gentle digital pressure. Too much pressure will obscure the pulse.

Pressure quality can be evaluated using one side, but a more thorough evaluation includes evaluation of bilateral femoral pulses. This is good practice because arterial thrombosis can impede one femoral arterial pulse and not the other.

Patients that present in hypovolemic states exhibit alteration in their pulse pressure. As previously discussed, when blood volume is diminished, less blood returns to the heart and CO decreases. If the heart is pumping less blood into the arteries, it makes sense that the associated arterial pulses will be appreciably weaker. Consequently, hypovolemic animals typically have pulses that are described as weak or thready (Kaplan 1992). In severe cases, femoral pulses may be impossible to palpate.

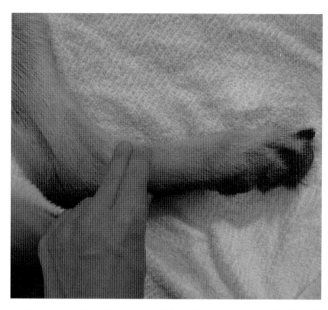

Figure 2.6. Dorsal pedal pulses are found on the cranial medial aspect of the hindfoot. The technician should become familiar with locating and palpating pulses at this location.

The technician must palpate femoral pulses in healthy as well as compromised patients to develop the ability to compare and accurately describe pulse quality.

Dorsal pedal (DP) pulses are often excluded from the initial physical assessment. At least one hind foot should be palpated to confirm the presence of DP pulses and to evaluate the strength of these pulses (Fig. 2.6).

DP pulses are usually the first pulses that disappear when an animal is hypovolemic. This is in part due to one of the body's compensatory mechanisms. In states of diminished circulating blood volume, the heart, brain, and kidneys are prioritized above all other organs and tissues (Wingfield 2002b). Because the peripheral limbs do not have a vital role in sustaining life, circulation is routed away from them toward higher priority areas. Lower blood circulation to these limbs causes DP pulses to be weak. Once again, in severe cases, DP pulses are absent. It has been suggested that DP pulses disappear at a mean arterial pressure (MAP) of approximately 60 mm Hg or when hypovolemia is so severe that the animal can no longer compensate (Wingfield 2002a).

Quick assessment tests

Part of the initial patient assessment includes collecting data such as vital parameters and various blood chemistries. Quick analysis tests (QUATS) are tests that can be run at cage side and provide preliminary information pertaining to the patient's hydration and volume status. Specific tests included in QUATS differ between hospitals depending on availability of equipment and personnel. An example of QUATS performed in a high-volume emergency and critical care setting might include packed cell volume (PCV) and total solids (TS), blood urea nitrogen (BUN) stick, blood glucose (BG), venous blood gases, electrolytes, blood lactate, and activated clotting time. In a lower volume hospital QUATS might be restricted to PCV/TS, BG, and BUN stick because routine health checks do not necessarily need to include such extensive QUATS as those previously listed. Results from each test can provide additional evidence to support findings of the initial physical assessment.

Packed cell volume

PCV refers to the percentage of intravascular fluid that is occupied by red blood cells. In varying degrees of illness PCV can deviate in either direction. Interpretation of changes in PCV can provide information to support or refute estimates of patient hydration status developed during the initial physical examination. Evaluation of PCV in conjunction with TS is key to understanding the composition of fluid lost or gained.

Increases in PCV and TS

Increases in PCV can indicate several conditions. The condition most relevant to this section is dehydration. A dehydrated patient often displays an elevated PCV in conjunction with an elevation of TS at the time of presentation (Fig. 2.7).

Excessive water loss from the extracellular compartment disturbs the fine balance of water throughout the body. For example, an animal that is vomiting or experiencing diarrhea loses excess body water from its extracellular compartment. The intravascular space is included in this compartment. Ongoing losses of this kind lead to depletion of water, causing the intravascular space to become hypertonic. Another way to perceive this change in balance is to consider that water is borrowed from the intracellular space in times of desperate need in the extracellular compartment (DiBartola 2006). As the condition or illness persists, less body water is available to maintain the volume of the extracellular space. This leads to a change in solute concentration of that compartment.

Depletion of water from the intravascular space, which is part of the extracellular compartment, causes hemoconcentration. The ratio between water, red blood cells, and

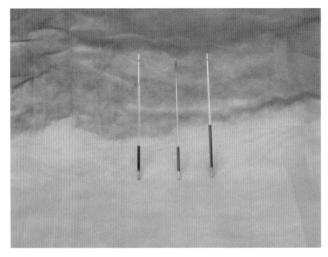

Figure 2.7. PCV tubes: Assessing PCV is an important part of the initial physical examination. Interpretation of PCV results can offer valuable information that contributes to the determination of patient hydration status.

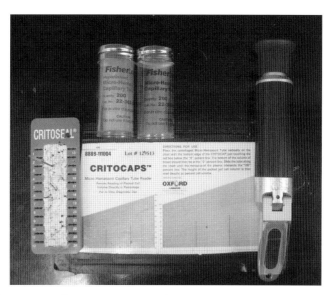

Figure 2.8. Supplies necessary for measuring PCV and TS.

plasma proteins (TS) is changed. The concentration of red blood cells and proteins circulating in intravascular fluid increases because the overall fluid volume is smaller.

Increased PCV and decreased TS

An increase in PCV in conjunction with a decrease in TS can be interpreted slightly differently than the previous example. A TS that is lower than normal in the face of an elevated PCV is likely an indication of pathology involving protein loss.

Decreased PCV and TS

Many forms of illness cause anemia. To provide appropriate therapy for anemic patients we must determine what is causing a decrease in PCV. Accurate interpretation of a decreased PCV also involves consideration of TS (Fig. 2.8).

A decreased PCV in conjunction with decreased TS is most often representative of whole blood loss (DiBartola 2006). A trauma patient has likely sustained damage to blood vessels and/or organs. A compromise to the integrity of a blood vessel leads to some degree of blood loss. It is the entire blood component that is lost from either of these compartments; not just red blood cells (RBCs) or proteins. So we note a decrease in both PCV and TS.

Decreases in PCV and TS may not be evident immediately post hemorrhage because the redistribution of fluids takes time to manifest. In addition, PCV may appear slightly elevated while TS remains low if the patient's spleen has contracted in an effort to compensate for the blood loss (Mathews 2006b).

In the face of blood loss the initial goal of fluid therapy is to replace the volume lost from the intravascular compartment. Serial measurements of PCV/TS are not as helpful in guiding fluid therapy protocols as they are in the dehydrated patient because these values are affected by so many other factors. For example, ongoing loss of blood, splenic contraction, and infusion of natural or synthetic colloids each cause changes in PCV or

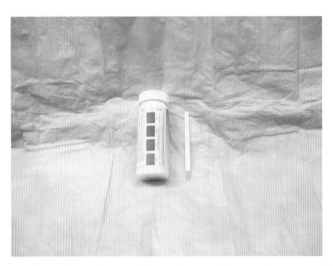

Figure 2.9. The BUN stick is a fast and easy test that can be run using a small amount of blood. These results aid in determining hydration status.

TS, respectively (DiBartola 2006). Rather, the therapy is guided by evaluation of volume status and should focus on BP, HR, MM color, and perfusion. This type of monitoring is discussed in greater detail in Chapter 6.

A decrease in PCV/TS may be appreciated in patients that have received fluid therapy. The patient that initially presents with elevated PCV/TS due to dehydration will likely display a drop in *both* of these values once rehydrated. It is important to note that an initial drop in values that coincides with initiation of fluid therapy is not indicative of blood loss. Continued or significant decreases in PCV/TS that extend beyond the point of rehydration should be investigated.

Blood urea nitrogen stick

This form of test is simple and convenient and available to most veterinary practices (Fig. 2.9). A small drop of whole blood is placed on a reagent strip for a set amount of time (usually 60 seconds). At the end of the prescribed time period the blood is washed off and the color of the strip is compared with a number of colors on the container provided. Each color corresponds to a range of values of BUN. Evaluation of the BUN stick provides another valuable piece of information that is considered during evaluation of patient hydration status.

Urea is a waste product that ends up in the blood and is ultimately filtered by the kidneys. Some of the urea is excreted in the urine and some of it returns to the blood. Because urea is a solute found in the blood, a loss of body water is reflected by an increase in the concentration of urea. Abnormally high BUN results can indicate a host of disease processes; however, an increased concentration of urea can also be an indication of dehydration.

Many other factors can cause elevations and decreases in BUN. As with most other means of patient evaluation, BUN must be used in conjunction with other physical and clinical data to provide valuable information regarding patient hydration status.

Venous blood gases and electrolytes

An in-depth discussion of blood gases and electrolytes is beyond the scope of this text. Dehydrated and/or hypovolemic animals can display many different patterns in their blood gases, ranging from virtually normal to severe metabolic acidosis with respiratory compensation. Blood gas measurement is a very useful tool available for guidance of fluid therapy; however, there is no definitive result that is diagnostic for dehydration.

Lactate

Illness causing loss of body water can result in decreased perfusion if water loss is profound, such as that seen with protracted vomiting with or without diarrhea. As poor perfusion reduces delivery of oxygen and nutrients to the tissues, diminished oxygen results in an environment in which cells carry out their functions in a state of hypoxia. Under normal circumstances cellular metabolism takes place in aerobic as well as anaerobic conditions. In hypoxic states, there is a shift toward anaerobic metabolism. This change causes an increase in the amount of lactate produced. Lactate spills out of the cells and into the blood. The excess lactate overwhelms the liver and the kidneys, organs that are normally responsible for metabolizing, buffering, and excreting lactate. As lactate levels increase, blood pH decreases (Mathews 2006c).

Elevations in lactate do not exclusively indicate conditions involving loss of body water. However, it is frequently noted that patients presenting in dehydrated or hypovolemic states are also found to have lactate levels above normal.

Urine specific gravity

The urine specific gravity (USG) measurement is most informative if obtained before administration of fluids. It is not always possible to obtain a urine sample from a critically ill patient shortly after presentation; however, should urine become available, even the smallest volume can be used for measurement of USG.

Most forms of veterinary practices possess a refractometer as part of their standard equipment. This instrument provides a fast and accurate measurement of USG (Fig. 2.10).

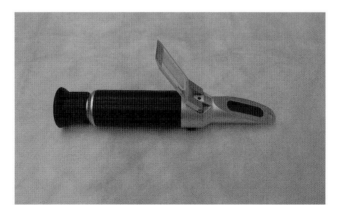

Figure 2.10. A refractometer is used to measure urine specific gravity.

Table 2.1   Range in Normal Blood Pressure Measurements

	Canine	Feline
Systolic	100–160 mm Hg	110–150 mm Hg
Diastolic	70–120 mm Hg	70–130 mm Hg
Mean Arterial Pressure (MAP)	80–120 mm Hg	100–150 mm Hg

Sources: McCurnin, D. *Clinical Textbook for Veterinary Technicians*, Saunders 1994; Wingfield, W. *The Veterinary ICU Book*, Teton NewMedia 2002; Wingfield, W. *Veterinary Emergency Medicine Secrets*, Hanley & Belfus 2001.

USG is a measurement of the concentration of solids in the urine. In health, the kidneys excrete a specific concentration of waste products that are filtered from the blood. In the dehydrated patient, the body attempts to conserve water by instructing healthy kidneys to excrete less urine. The volume of waste product does not change dramatically, which leads to a higher solute concentration in the smaller volume of urine excreted. Dehydrated patients possessing healthy kidneys present with a higher USG than animals in perfect health (DiBartola and Bateman 2006).

Blood pressure

BP monitoring is available to many technicians in emergency and critical care settings but may not yet be part of the standard of care in private primary care facilities. Its lack of availability in these settings does not dictate that technicians practicing in primary care clinics should not have at least a basic understanding of BP monitoring. Veterinary medicine is a perpetually growing field, and with the increasing availability of affordable equipment, it is likely that BP monitoring will become the standard for all clinics in the very near future. Two types of BP measurement are used in veterinary medicine: direct arterial BP measurement (also known as invasive monitoring) and indirect BP measurement (noninvasive monitoring). The invasive technique involves placement of an indwelling arterial catheter; noninvasive techniques rely on machine sensitivity and require less technical nursing. Equipment used for BP is discussed in Chapter 6.

The initial physical examination should include BP measurement where available. Despite how thorough the physical examination might be, there is always more information to be garnered from additional tests. BP helps tailor the earliest stage of fluid administration to each individual patient. BP has three components that are measured and recorded. Systolic BP refers to the pressure that exists in the arteries during the phase of cardiac contraction (systole). Diastolic BP refers to the pressure in the arteries during the rest phase of the cardiac cycle (diastole). The MAP is the average pressure throughout the cycle of the heart. Canine and feline patients display a range of blood pressures (in good health) that are accepted as normal (see Table 2.1). A MAP of 100, with a systolic/diastolic of 120/80 is a value that can be used for comparison because these numbers fall roughly in the middle of the acceptable range.

The technician can use the MAP to establish how immediately the patient requires medical intervention. MAP measurements of 70 mm Hg and below represent compromised tissue and organ perfusion (Hammond and Walters 1999). Patients with MAPs of 70 mm Hg or less need a greater degree of intervention and more intensive monitoring than those that present with near normal MAP values (≥80 mm Hg).

Case Studies

Administration of intravenous (IV) fluids is the core of intervention in critically ill patients. IV access is a priority that is only superseded by obtaining a patent airway and/or administering emergency drugs. The following cases illustrate the changes brought about through appropriate use of fluid therapy. Vitals were used at time of presentation to determine the immediacy of each patient's need for fluids. Once various volumes had been administered, vitals were used to reassess the patient's response to fluids and determine whether or not therapy should continue as prescribed.

Case 1

Signalment: 9-year-old male neutered standard poodle

Presented to hospital with history of anorexia, vomiting, lethargy, and two episodes of diarrhea. Upon admission physical examination revealed the following:

- Body weight: 29.7 kg
- Temperature: 40.0°C
- Pulse: 210 beats per minute (bpm)
- Pulse quality strong
- Respiratory rate: panting
- MMs: pink, tacky
- Capillary refill time (CRT): <2 seconds
- BP: 140/84; MAP: 106
- Lactate: 5.3 mmol/L

 Nursing considerations

Tachycardia, elevated body temperature, and elevated lactate are of most concern in this patient. Many factors could be responsible for each of these abnormalities. Based on the patient's elevated lactate and elevated HR, it was determined that his perfusion was compromised.

Initial intervention included a fluid bolus of 10 mL/kg (300 mL) IV Plasmalyte A given over 15 minutes. The patient's vitals were reevaluated after the first fluid bolus and reflected a significant improvement in HR (120 bpm). BP also changed but remained within normal limits before and after fluid bolus. It is interesting to note that after IV administration of 300 mL of crystalloid fluids, the patient's BP increased from 140/84 MAP of 106 to 166/94 MAP 116. Many factors may have contributed to this increase (fear, pain, anxiety), but it is also likely that increasing the circulating blood volume with a fluid bolus played a role in instigating this change in BP.

Upon completion of the fluid bolus the patient was placed on IV fluids at two times maintenance rate. Three hours after admission his body temperature had also improved significantly and had decreased from 40.0°C to 38.1°C. Febrile patients have additional fluid requirements during rehydration. Once a fluid rate has been determined, an additional volume (0.1 × maintenance rate) should be added for each degree Celsius that the patient measures above normal (38.5°C) (Mathews 2006a).

Lactate measurement was repeated 8 hours after commencement of fluid therapy and had decreased to 3.0 mmol/L. An additional 12 hours of fluid therapy resulted in a decrease to a lactate of 1.8 mmol/L, which is within normal limits.

Improvement in each of these parameters was a direct result of fluid administration. The early stages of fluid therapy led to an increase in intravascular volume and a decrease in heart rate (fewer beats needed to achieve similar CO once intravascular volume had increased). Once the patient was placed on a moderate rate of continuous IV fluids, his body temperature began to normalize. Perhaps the most impressive change brought about with this fluid therapy was the normalization of the patient's lactate. Improved perfusion allows appropriate delivery of oxygenated blood to the cells. Improving this patient's perfusion meant that the cells were no longer functioning in anaerobic conditions, thus producing less lactate.

Case 2

Signalment: 2-year-old male neutered dachshund

Presented with a history of hemorrhagic vomiting of approximately 12 hours duration. The owner also noted blood in the dog's stool. On presentation to the referring veterinarian the dog was found to have the following vitals:

■ Quiet, alert, and responsive
■ HR: 108 bpm
■ Respiratory rate: 42 breaths per minute
■ MMs: pale pink, moist with prolonged (>2 seconds) CRT
■ Extremities: cool

The initial blood work revealed an elevated RBC count (10.3×10^{12}/L) (normal: $5.5–8.5 \times 10^{12}$/L); elevated packed cell volume 67.8% (normal: 37%–55%); elevated hemoglobin 212 g/L (normal: 133–197 g/L). The patient received a 10 mL/kg IV bolus of Plasmalyte over 15 minutes. Repeat examination post fluid bolus revealed improvement in peripheral perfusion. The dog's MMs were a deeper pink, the extremities were thought to be warmer, and the dog's CRT was <2 seconds. The referring veterinarian evaluated the patient and felt that he was stable enough to transfer to a tertiary care facility.

The patient presented to the referral hospital approximately 2 hours after initial arrival at his regular veterinarian. He had the following vitals:

■ HR: 144 bpm
■ Respiratory rate: 32 breaths per minute
■ MMs: pink and tacky
■ CRT: 2 seconds
■ Temperature: 37.9°C
■ Slightly prolonged skin tent
■ Blood pressure: 151/61; MAP 101
■ Estimated dehydration: 7%

Initial blood work revealed a PCV of 65% (normal: 37%–55%); TS of 62 g/L (60–80 g/L); lactate of 2.2 mmol/L (normal <2 mmol/L); and BUN stick: 30 to 40 mg/dL (normal <15 mg/dL).

 Nursing considerations

Tachycardia, tacky MMs, and prolonged skin tent are of concern in this patient. After reviewing the patient's blood work, polycythemia (elevated PCV), mildly elevated lactate, and elevated BUN are of further concern. Despite initial intervention by the referring veterinarian, these findings point toward the conclusion that this patient is dehydrated.

The patient received a 20 mL/kg IV fluid bolus of 0.9% NaCl over 30 minutes. Blood gases showed that he was mildly alkalemic, which prompted the use of an acidifying solution (NaCl). After the bolus, the patient was started on a continuous IV infusion of 0.9% NaCl at two times maintenance rate for 6 hours. Vitals and QUATS were reevaluated after the initial 6 hours of fluids and showed improvement.

Heart rate had decreased to 96 bpm, MMs were pink and moist, CRT was <2 seconds, lactate decreased to 1.0 mmol/L, BUN stick decreased to 5 to 15 mg/dL, PCV/TS decreased to 53/4.0, and BP was mildly elevated at 178/60; MAP 116.

The fluid therapy prescription was changed in response to the vitals. The patient's low total solids were of particular concern and a colloid infusion (Pentaspan) was added to provide oncotic support to the intravascular space. Crystalloid therapy was changed from 0.9% NaCl to Plasmalyte A because the patient's metabolic alkalosis had resolved.

Chapter Summary

The main focus of this chapter has revolved around the effects of body water loss and how they are detected during the physical examination. Recall that dehydration is a condition that involves an overall loss of body water in excess of what the patient is able to replace. Most water loss occurs in the intracellular and interstitial compartments.

A patient's hydration status should be evaluated during the technician's primary survey. Tacky or dry MMs are frequently noted in the dehydrated patient. Sunken eye position, prolonged skin tent, and mild changes in mentation are also signs that a patient is suffering from some degree of dehydration.

Hypovolemia refers to a decreased volume of fluid circulating within the vasculature. This condition leads to poor perfusion and puts vital organs and tissues at great risk as a result.

Many veterinary patients suffer from dehydration and hypovolemia simultaneously. Each condition can exist independent of the other and each can be life threatening if left untreated.

A primary survey examination includes vital parameters that are useful in determining whether or not a patient is hypovolemic. Volume-depleted patients present with an elevated HR, decreased pulse amplitude, weak or thready pulses, and possibly a prolonged CRT. Initial lab work often reveals elevated PCV and TS; elevated BUN stick; elevated lactate, and elevated USG.

Review Questions

1. Define hypovolemia.
2. List three parameters easily evaluated by the technician at the time of patient admission that may reveal the hydration status of the animal.
3. How does hypovolemia affect cardiac output?
4. In the face of hypovolemia, the body benefits from the activation of its natural protective mechanisms. Ultimately, what is the goal of these protective measures?
5. Why is it prudent to palpate femoral pulses on both hind limbs?
6. If dorsal pedal pulses are not palpable to the experienced technician, what assumptions can be made with respect to the patient's status?
7. An elevated PCV/TS can indicate that the patient is (a)_____, whereas an elevated PCV and decreased TS could indicate (b)_____. (c) However, normal to elevated PCV and low TS in the face of recent hemorrhage is also possible. Why is this?
8. A dehydrated animal with normal renal function should excrete urine with a (a)_____ urine specific gravity (USG). (b) Why is this the case?

Answers to the review questions can be found on pages 221–222 in the Appendix. The review questions are also available for download on a companion website at www.wiley. com/go/donohoenursing.

Further Reading

Cooper, E., and W. Muir. 2007. Continuous cardiac output monitoring via arterial pressure waveform analysis following severe hemorrhagic shock in dogs. *Crit Care Med* 35:1724–1729.

DiBartola, S., and S. Bateman. 2006. Introduction to fluid therapy. In S. DiBartola, ed. *Fluid, Electrolyte, and Acid Base Disorders in Small Animal Practice*, 325–344. St. Louis: Saunders.

DiBartola, S. 2006. Disorders of sodium and water: hypernatremia and hyponatremia. In S. DiBartola, ed. *Fluid, Electrolyte, and Acid Base Disorders in Small Animal Practice*, 47–79. St. Louis: Saunders.

Hammond, R., and C. Walters. 1999. Monitoring the critical patient. In L.G. King, ed. *Manual of Canine and Feline Emergency and Critical Care*, 235–246. Cheltenham, UK: BSAVA.

Hughes, D. 1999. Fluid therapy. In L.G. King, *Manual of Canine and Feline Emergency and Critical Care*, 7–22. Cheltenham, UK: BSAVA.

Kaplan, P. 1992. *Monitoring in Veterinary Emergency and Critical Care Medicine*, 21–37. St. Louis: Mosby.

King, L., and R. Hammond. 1999. *Manual of Canine and Feline Emergency and Critical Care*. Cheltenham, UK: BSAVA.

Mathews, K. 1998. The various types of parenteral fluids and their indications. *Vet Clin North Am Small Anim Pract* 28:489–490.

Mathews, K. 2006a. Fluid therapy: non-hemorrhage. In K. Mathews, ed. *Veterinary Emergency and Critical Care Manual*, 347–373. Guelph, Ontario, Canada: LifeLearn.

Mathews, K. 2006b. Hemorrhage. In K. Mathews, ed. *Veterinary Emergency and Critical Care Manual*, 619–629. Guelph, Ontario, Canada: LifeLearn.

Mathews, K. 2006c. Lactate. In K. Mathews, ed. *Veterinary Emergency and Critical Care Manual*, 400–405. Guelph, Ontario, Canada: LifeLearn.

Mensack, S. 2008. Fluid therapy: options and rational administration. *Vet Clin North Am Small Anim Pract* 38:575–577.

Miller, C. 2002. Applied cardiovascular physiology. In W.E. Wingfield and M. R. Raffe, eds., *The Veterinary ICU Book*, 1–14. Jackson, WY: Teton NewMedia.

Miller, M., S. DiBartola, and E. Schertel. 1992. Conventional and hypertonic fluid therapy: concepts and applications. In R.J. Murtaugh, ed. *Veterinary Emergency and Critical Care Medicine*, 618–627. St. Louis: Mosby.

Peitzman, A. 1993. Hypovolemic shock. In M. Pinsky and J. Dhainaut, eds. *Pathophysiologic Foundations of Critical Care*, 161–169. Baltimore: Williams & Wilkins.

Wingfield, W.E. 2002a. Cardiopulmonary arrest. In W.E. Wingfield and M. R. Raffe, eds., *The Veterinary ICU Book*, 421–452. Jackson, WY: Teton NewMedia.

Wingfield, W.E. 2002b. Fluid and electrolyte therapy. In W.E. Wingfield and M. R. Raffe, eds., *The Veterinary ICU Book*, 166–188. Jackson, WY: Teton NewMedia.

Routes of Administration

3

Fluid therapy is administered in many different settings throughout the practice of veterinary medicine. The means by which fluids are delivered must be selected based on a variety of factors. It is helpful to know the anticipated duration of fluid therapy, the patient's current hydration/volume status, the patient's current health concerns, and the patient's approachability before determining the ideal route for fluid administration. With this information the health care team can decide on the safest, most efficient route for delivery of fluids.

Gastrointestinal Tract (Enteral Fluid Administration)

The enteral route is often overlooked as a potential path for fluid therapy. This is likely due to the fact that many of our patients requiring fluid therapy are exhibiting clinical signs that involve some form of disruption in their gastrointestinal (GI) health. Animals whose history includes episodes of vomiting, diarrhea, abdominal distention, esophageal trauma, or decrease of esophageal motility will not tolerate fluid therapy via the enteral route. If GI health is without compromise, enteral fluid therapy may be considered for patients with mild disturbances in their hydration or volume status. In other words, if it is appropriate to replace fluid deficits slowly, the enteral route is a suitable choice. In contrast, if the patient is suffering from severe blood loss or acute hemorrhage, the enteral route is not a suitable route for volume resuscitation. This is because fluid delivered to the GI tract would require too much time to redistribute and replenish the intravascular space.

Fluid Therapy for Veterinary Technicians and Nurses, First Edition. Charlotte Donohoe.
© 2012 Charlotte Donohoe. Published 2012 by John Wiley & Sons, Inc.

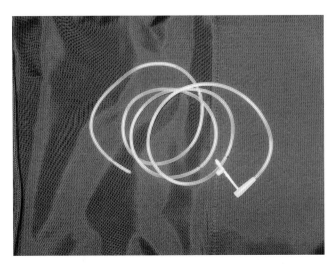

Figure 3.1. This type of tube can be used as a nasoesophageal feeding tube. The tube is a worthwhile inventory item because it can also be used as a nasal oxygen catheter or canine male urinary catheter.

Benefits associated with enteral fluid therapy include the potential for delivery of large volumes of fluid as well as delivery of fluids with a variety of caloric densities. If caloric support is not a concern, the clinician should choose a maintenance fluid that is similar to the extracellular compartment with respect to solute concentration. The fluid may contain dextrose (2.5%–5%) that aids absorption and can help prepare the patient for enteral feeding that may play a role in the therapeutic plan.

Patients that are not voluntarily ingesting liquids may be candidates for placement of one of a variety of different feeding tubes. Tubes can be placed using mild to moderate sedation or general anesthesia depending on the type of tube required. In most cases, clinicians place enteral feeding tubes such as esophagostomy and percutaneous gastrostomy tubes. However, the veterinary technician is trained in and responsible for delivery of fluids as well as care and maintenance of tubes for the duration of their dwell.

Nasoesophageal Feeding Tubes

Nasoesophageal feeding tubes (NE tubes) are flexible plastic or rubber tubes that are passed into the esophagus via the patient's nose (Fig. 3.1). These tubes are relatively easy to place and are most often placed and secured by the technician. A variety of types of tubes are available, which allows the technician to select an appropriate length and diameter for each patient. The tube should fit with relative ease into the opening of the ventral meatus but should not be markedly smaller than its diameter. The length of the tube must allow for its passage beyond the nasopharynx and into the esophagus. A tube that is too short will not permit passage far enough into the esophagus. In contrast, a tube that offers excessive length may still be used providing the excess is safely and securely fastened *on* rather than *in* the patient.

The technician should have all necessary materials within reach before beginning the placement procedure. In most cases the patient would prefer not to undergo NE tube placement, and for this reason the technician must perform the procedure quickly and efficiently. Scrambling for materials mid-placement lengthens the process, stresses the patient and technician, and typically prevents successful positioning of the tube.

The patient's nose can be numbed with a topical anesthetic (ophthalmic drops work well) approximately 10 to 15 minutes before beginning. It is advisable to place drops in both nostrils in the event that the first attempt does not result in successful placement of the tube. In some patients one side provides easier access than the other. Having both nostrils prepared with drops allows efficient use of the technician's time and avoids a wait once in the midst of the procedure.

NE tubes must be measured before placement to ensure the fluid is delivered to the desired location (the esophagus). The tube is measured by holding it against the patient's body and determining the length of tube needed to extend the tube from the seventh intercostal space to the tip of the nose. The tube should be held with the open end (connection port) distal to the patient and the closed delivery end at the location of the seventh intercostal space. In so doing, a permanent marker can be used to draw a small line on the tube where it reaches the level of the tip of the nose. The tube can then be passed using the level of the black mark as a guideline for depth of placement. Once the tube is measured, the proximal end can be lightly lubricated with an oral anesthetic such as 2% viscous lidocaine gel. Only a thin layer of lidocaine gel is necessary to facilitate smooth introduction of the tube.

The tube is placed in the nostril and guided in a ventromedial direction to enter the ventral meatus. The tube should encounter little to no resistance if advancing along the correct path. In some patients it is possible to observe a swallowing reflex as the tube passes through the larynx. This event is not witnessed in every instance.

Once the tube is advancing well, the technician can use the measured mark on the tube as a reference point at which to stop advancing. Once the mark is at the distal end of the rostrum, the tube has advanced far enough. The tube can be secured to the patient's face using a number of different methods. In the author's experience, sutures or tiny drops (pinpoint size) of Krazy Glue™ are the most successful way to secure the tube.

Proper placement of the tube must be confirmed before using the NE tube for fluid therapy or delivery of nutrition. This is accomplished with a series of actions. First, the technician can attach a 5-mL syringe to the port of the tube and apply gentle negative pressure. If the tube is in the esophagus, the negative pressure should remain relatively constant and the aspiration should yield no fluid. If negative pressure is achieved, the tube can be withdrawn 2 to 3 cm and negative pressure reapplied. The rationale for repositioning the tube is to rule out the possibility of bronchial placement of the tube. Negative pressure will remain constant if the tube is in the esophagus and not the lower airway.

If aspiration continuously yields air, it is likely that the tube has been placed incorrectly and is in the trachea. A radiograph is useful to verify the tube's location. If there is any uncertainty at all, the tube should be removed and the procedure repeated.

If the initial or subsequent aspirations suggest correct placement (negative pressure), a small volume of sterile saline is injected into the tube. The patient is closely observed for any sign of discomfort or distress associated with the delivery of fluid through the tube. Placement of the NE tube in the patient's airway normally leads to moderate amounts of coughing once the saline has been injected. If the patient swallows or licks the lips when saline is injected and does not cough, the tube is likely in the correct location.

A radiograph of the patient's cranial thorax can corroborate correct placement of the NE tube.

Complications are infrequent with NE tubes. If complications do arise, they are usually among the following:

- Tracheal intubation due to difficulty with placement
- Vomiting leads to removal of tube and/or animal chews tube once it has been vomited into mouth
- Mild nasal discharge or rhinitis may be seen in animals with NE tube in place for prolonged period of time

Nursing considerations

- NE feeding tubes can be used for continuous delivery of fluids or intermittent boluses of fluids
- NE tubes are not an appropriate selection for patients that are vomiting or regurgitating
- NE tubes should not be used in patients that are semi or unconscious
- Patients can eat or drink with NE tubes in place if desired

Esophagostomy and Gastrostomy Feeding Tubes

The esophagostomy and gastrostomy tubes are most often reserved for patients that require long-term support (Fig. 3.2A–C). In addition, they are a more likely choice for patients that require nutritional support, in clinic or at home, rather than patients that require fluid therapy alone. Supplemental fluids can also be delivered via esophagostomy or gastrostomy tube to patients that are receiving fluid therapy via other routes.

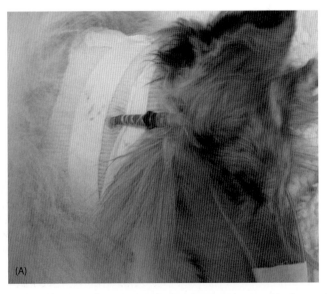

(A)

Figure 3.2.   (A) A patient with an esophagostomy tube bandaged and secured in the cervical region.

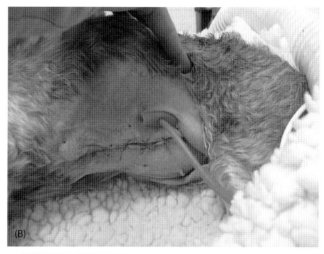

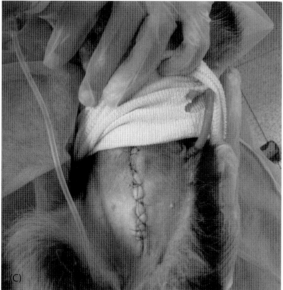

Figure 3.2. *(Continued)* (B) Gastrostomy tubes can be used in animals that are unable to tolerate feeding in their upper gastrointestinal tract. (C) Gastrostomy tube location with body sleeve to reduce contamination of tube stoma.

The clinician places these tubes, but they are monitored by the technician. Because these tubes are used in most tertiary care hospitals, much information is available with respect to surgical placement of tubes. See the suggested reading section for procedural information.

Tube care is simple but is an important contribution to the comfort of the patient. Each of these tubes involves a stoma that must be kept clean and free of external debris. The stoma should be monitored for signs of discharge, excessive swelling, or excessive redness. The site should be cleaned daily or every other day with warm water and gauze.

The esophagostomy tube stoma is bandaged using a layer of padding, such as Conform (Kendall) or Protouch Plus (synthetic orthopedic padding, BSN Medical), and a wrap such as Vetrap (3M) as the outer layer. Gastrostomy tubes can be covered with an elasticized stockinette such as Protouch Cotton Stockinette (BSN Medical). This product is an expandable cotton-blend material that can be cut into a T-shirt of sorts. The stockinette is doubled and an additional hole is made in the first layer to allow the tube to sit between the two layers of material. This keeps dirt and debris off of the tube and away from the stoma while keeping the tube fairly low profile to avoid accidental removal.

The tubes should be securely capped with an appropriate adapter whenever they are not connected to continuous infusions. Otherwise, the technician should evaluate the connection site and fluid infusion set for cleanliness and replace as needed.

Subcutaneous Fluid Administration

Subcutaneous (SC) administration of fluids is widely used in small animal medicine. It is a practical means by which fluids can be delivered to noncritical patients. Advantages to SC administration include low cost, decreased demand for advanced technical skills, improved patient acceptance, and lack of need for hospitalization. Feline and small canine patients experiencing mild dehydration may be treated with SC fluids and discharged in the care of their owners, which makes SC fluid therapy an attractive option for clients. This route can be used with a moderate degree of safety providing that the patient does not have any underlying cardiac disease.

Limitations to SC fluid administration include the volume of fluid that can be administered to a patient at one time. Each SC site can tolerate approximately 10 mL/kg of fluid. More than one site can be used per patient per visit, but the patient's comfort is compromised when he or she is laden with multiple sites of SC fluid administration.

Fluids are administered along the dorsum of the animal's body between the scapulae and lower lumbar vertebrae. Given the restricted area for administration, it is common for a patient to receive between one and three boluses of SC fluids at a time.

The practice of SC fluid administration varies between veterinary hospitals. Several guidelines should be considered when using this style of fluid therapy. For example, not all fluids can safely be delivered into the SC space. Fluids containing dextrose or high concentrations of potassium (K+) are not suitable. Fluids containing a concentration of up to 30 mEq/L of K+ can be used (DiBartola and Bateman 2006). Delivery of isotonic fluids is required; lactated Ringer's solution and normal saline (0.9% NaCl) are well tolerated in most patients. Increased patient comfort is achieved by warming fluids to body temperature when possible. In addition, administration of warm fluids can improve blood flow to the area and expedite absorption of fluids as a result.

It is acceptable to deliver SC fluids via needle and syringe; however, administration using a sterile bag of fluids with a drip set and needle is safer. The needle and syringe method requires that the fluids be delivered under pressure while the solution set allows fluids to flow into SC space using the force of gravity. Although the skin and subcutaneous tissue adapt to the presence of the fluid volume with time, faster delivery via syringe forces the fluid volume into a confined space that is less forgiving without the benefit of time (DiBartola and Bateman 2006).

An 18- to 20-gauge needle is suitable for most patients, but very small patients may require a 22-gauge needle to achieve cooperation. Ideally the needle is attached to a sterile administration set and a new bag of intravenous (IV) fluids. The administration set can be either a macro drip or micro drip. A macro drip delivers the same volume of fluid in a shorter time than the micro drip.

Despite the safety and usefulness of SC fluid administration, there are circumstances during which this type of therapy is contraindicated.

SC fluid therapy relies on the peripheral tissue to absorb and carry fluid to the vasculature. If blood flow to peripheral vessels is compromised, the absorption of the fluid is slow and distribution of the fluid to the rest of the body is diminished (Mensack 2008). For this reason patients that are severely hypotensive, markedly dehydrated, or hypothermic are not candidates for SC fluid therapy.

Intraperitoneal Fluid Administration

The peritoneum is the layer of serosa that lines the abdominal cavity and covers the organs within the abdomen. The peritoneal membrane is divided into two sections. The parietal peritoneum lines the inner wall of the abdomen. The visceral peritoneum covers the organs that lie within this compartment. The two sections are continuous and joined by the connecting peritoneum. The kidneys are found outside of the peritoneal membrane and are thus described as retroperitoneal organs.

The peritoneal cavity is the area that lies between parietal and visceral peritoneum. It contains a small volume of fluid that serves as lubrication between the two serosal layers. No organs are housed within the peritoneal cavity.

Intraperitoneal (IP) fluid administration involves delivery of fluids into the peritoneal cavity. IP fluid administration is not a routine procedure in current veterinary practice. However, there are some benefits to this route if no other is available. Given the relative size of the peritoneal space, a moderate volume of fluids can be delivered without compromise to patient comfort. Fluid is absorbed from the peritoneal cavity over approximately 24 to 48 hours (Ogg 2003). This lengthy time of absorption makes IP fluid therapy inappropriate for patients experiencing hypovolemic shock. Pediatric patients may be an exception to this in the event that venous access is unobtainable. It is necessary to use isotonic fluids for delivery into the peritoneal cavity to avoid causing unwanted fluid shifts.

Strict aseptic technique is mandatory when introducing a catheter into the peritoneal cavity. Introduction of bacteria can cause moderate to severe inflammation. Peritonitis is a condition involving swelling of the peritoneum. It is an extremely painful condition that is also life threatening. Given that peritonitis is a possible complication associated with IP fluid therapy, this route is not routinely recommended in veterinary patients (DiBartola and Bateman 2006).

Intraosseous Fluid Administration

Intraosseous (IO) fluid administration is extremely useful in veterinary medicine. Fluid delivery is achieved via a catheter or needle inserted into the marrow of select long bones. The intraosseous space is structurally stable and provides a compartment whose accessibility does not change in times of compromised health. Whereas vascular access can be difficult to obtain in a cardiovascularly collapsed patient, the shape and size of the intramedullary space does not vary in response to a patient's volume status. For this reason, IO fluid administration is an excellent alternative to IV fluid therapy in hypovolemic or dehydrated patients. IO catheterization and fluid delivery can also be achieved in very small or neonatal patients in whom vascular access is unobtainable.

A distinct advantage to IO fluid administration is the quick redistribution of fluids. Movement of IO fluid has been compared with delivery of fluid into the proximal vena cava (Gelens 2003). The volume and rate of fluid administration is similar to that encountered with IV fluid therapy. The rate at which fluids flow through a catheter is determined by the diameter of the catheter itself. A catheter with a large diameter and short length is appropriate for rapid administration of fluids. The diameter of the inside of the catheter is ultimately what determines the maximum rate at which the fluids will flow (Waddell 2004).

In addition to catheter diameter, catheter position can affect the flow rate of IO fluids. If the IO catheter is positioned right against the wall of the cortex, fluids may not flow freely into the marrow. If the catheter takes up bony material within its lumen during placement, it may become occluded.

Complications may arise but are uncommon with the IO route of administration. Pain during placement of the catheter is a common finding. The periosteum is very sensitive and should be locally anesthetized before placement. Patient discomfort is also a concern with elevated fluid rates. Flow by gravity is believed to be more comfortable. IO fluids can be warmed to improve patient comfort (Wingfield 2002a). An additional complication of concern using IO catheters is damage to regional nerves. Incorrect placement can lead to catheter-induced trauma to nerves (Mathews 2006).

Further complications, such as osteomyelitis, can arise if strict aseptic technique is not followed. It is an infrequent but serious complication associated with IO fluid therapy. Another potential complication with this route of fluid delivery is that personnel may have difficulty identifying landmarks (Olsen et al. 2002).

The trochanteric fossa of the femur, the greater tubercle of the humerus, and the tibial tuberosity are the most widely used sites for IO access (Figs. 3.3 and 3.4). Limbs affected

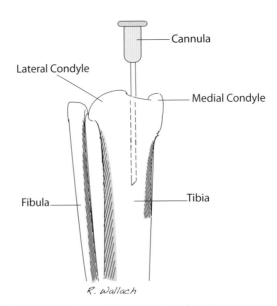

Figure 3.3. Intraosseous catheters can be used for patients in whom intravenous access is unobtainable. The tibial tuberosity is one of the preferred locations. Illustration by Rachel Wallach.

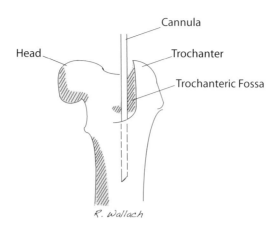

Figure 3.4. The trochanteric fossa of the femur is another choice location for an intraosseous catheter. Illustration by Rachel Wallach.

by trauma, infection, or pathologic fracture are inappropriate sites for IO fluid administration.

Once the site has been selected, the surrounding area should be generously clipped and surgically prepared. The periosteum is numbed by injection of approximately 1 mL of 1% or 2% lidocaine (DiBartola and Bateman 2006). A spinal needle, a hypodermic needle, or an IO catheter can be used for fluid administration. The catheter is inserted into the medulla in the direction of the long axis of the bone. A gentle rotation can be used in conjunction with the application of pressure in order to pass the needle or catheter into the marrow. The catheter should be passed up to the hub, so the hub is seated on the surface of the skin. The patency and appropriate placement of the catheter can be confirmed using a slow injection of heparinized saline flush (1 IU heparin/1 mL 0.9% NaCl). The flush should flow with virtually no resistance.

Once proper placement has been established, the catheter can be secured using medical tape, padding, and standard catheter bandaging materials. The patient's comfort is an important consideration when securing the catheter. Padding to cushion the hub of the needle is ideal, but securing the catheter is of utmost importance.

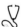 ## *Nursing considerations*

The tissue surrounding the bone should be evaluated as soon as continuous fluid infusion has begun. Further, routine investigation of the bandage and catheter site will alert the technician to any potential problems that may arise. Sites should be evaluated a minimum of once daily; twice daily is ideal.

Troubleshooting difficulties with IO catheters is similar to investigating IV catheters. Inappropriate positioning of the catheter can lead to interruption of flow. If the catheter is against the wall of the cortex, the needle can be rotated slightly so that the bevel is moved away from that surface.

Obstruction of flow can also be due to bone becoming lodged in the lumen of the catheter as it passes through the periosteum. This results in a bone plug. The plug can be removed by flushing with heparinized saline.

Fluids routinely delivered via IV therapy are acceptable for delivery through the IO route. Providing patient comfort is well established (with respect to IO catheter), this

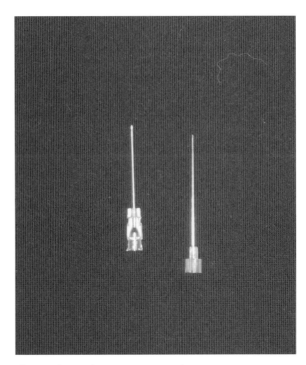

Figure 3.5. Spinal needles can be used as intraosseous catheters.

route can be used beyond the emergency phase of treatment. Typical use of the IO route is limited to between 12 and 24 hours. In many cases, it is used only until the point at which IV access is obtainable. Although uncommon, it is possible to administer fluids at an IO site for up to 3 days (Gelens 2003).

Several types of catheter-like devices are available for use in IO therapy. Selection is based on size and age of patient as well as availability of materials. Regardless of which style of catheter is chosen, a standard solution set can be connected to the hub and used for fluid administration.

Hypodermic needles are well suited as IO catheters in neonatal patients. Size varies with operator preference, but 18- to 20-gauge needles work well with most neonatal patients. Large or adult patients are better matched with spinal needles or IO catheters. The benefit of these two types of catheters is that they have a stylet. The presence of the stylet not only provides some rigidity to the catheter, but also prevents a bone plug from becoming lodged within the catheter. An additional advantage of IO catheters (commercially available) is that they have two opposing fenestrations at the proximal end of the catheter. This helps avoid obstruction of flow if the catheter is butted against the wall of the cortex.

Intravenous Fluid Administration

The IV route is widely accepted as the most useful and versatile means of administering fluid therapy to veterinary patients. Fluids can be delivered in large volumes and can be given expediently when necessary.

Hospitalized animals benefit from IV fluids during prophylactic, general health, and therapeutic procedures. One of the benefits to IV therapy is the degree to which it can be tailored to individual patients. A patient that is mildly dehydrated can receive replacement fluids delivered as a continuous rate infusion over a predetermined period of time; typically hours to days. There are many ways in which the clinician can determine the volume of fluids necessary for a given patient. The following is an example of one method of replacing the dehydration deficit (BW = body weight):

$$(BW) \times (\% \text{ dehydration}) \times (1000)$$

= Volume to be delivered to patient: half as bolus over 15 to 30 minutes;

half as replacement over 12 to 24 hours (Wingfield 2002b)

Severely volume depleted patients that present in shock may require immediate volume support, which can be achieved by administering an IV bolus of fluids. Fluid boluses are frequently delivered to patients during the emergency phase of treatment. The patient must be closely monitored for its response to each bolus. Careful attention is paid to all of the patient's vital parameters. Serial thoracic auscultations must be included in the monitoring to ensure no sudden changes develop with respect to lung sounds.

The IV route is also useful as a means of replacing fluid deficits, replacing ongoing losses, and providing maintenance fluids to patients that cannot meet their fluid needs independently.

This method allows for delivery of a variety of different types of fluids. Crystalloids, natural and synthetic colloids, blood products, cytotoxic (chemotherapeutic) drugs, and parenteral nutrition can all be delivered IV. Many pharmaceutical products used in veterinary therapy are available for IV use. The benefit of giving medications via the IV route is that repeated delivery does not require that the animal be injected each time the medication is given. Medications can be injected into the ports on delivery sets and infused *slowly* with fluid administration. Aseptic technique is mandatory for each puncture of the injection ports. IV catheters are available in several different styles, diameters, and lengths.

Nursing considerations

IV delivery of fluids should not be undertaken without recognition of potential complications. Although current techniques allow for very safe and successful use of this route, improper care of IV delivery systems and fluids can be detrimental to the patient. Failure to use strict aseptic technique during placement of catheters, as well as during setup of fluid bags, syringes, and associated equipment, can lead to inflammation and/or infection at the catheter site. Phlebitis is also a potential problem associated with use of improper technique.

While deciding whether or not to provide IV therapy to a patient, the veterinary team must consider if it is appropriate to do so in their specific clinical setting. Patients receiving IV fluids require constant and sometimes intensive monitoring. Therapy can be equipment intensive as well: Catheter supplies, infusion sets, infusion pumps, monitoring equipment, and technical personnel are but a few of the necessary tools.

Placement of the IV catheter is one of the cornerstones of fluid therapy. This is a skill that should largely be the responsibility of the technician. Catheter size, material, style, and location are selected based on patient species, size, and health requirements.

Intravenous Catheters

The frequent use of IV fluid therapy in humans has provided the veterinary medical community with many different types of catheters. Catheter size is determined by the measurement of the outer diameter of the cannula. Size is described as catheter gauge. There is an inverse relationship between catheter gauge and diameter size. Larger gauges correspond to smaller diameter cannulas; smaller gauges correspond to larger diameter cannulas. IV catheters are available in a range of sizes. Catheter diameters most commonly used in small animal practice typically fall between 24 and 14 gauges. Catheter diameter is an important aspect of IV fluid therapy because there is a direct relationship between the rate at which fluids will flow and the inner diameter of the catheter. According to this relationship, high rates of fluids are most appropriately administered via a large diameter (small gauge) catheter (Waddell 2004).

Catheters are also available in different lengths. Selection should be based on patient anatomy, the location of catheter placement, and the intended use. Patients with long limbs can comfortably house longer catheters in peripheral veins. Shorter catheters are appropriate for smaller patients or for those that have disproportionately short limbs.

Long catheters placed in the jugular vein may reach the cranial vena cava. Long catheters placed in the medial or lateral saphenous veins may reach the caudal vena cava. These catheters are termed *central venous catheters* or *central lines*.

IV catheters are available in different materials. The material can contribute to associated complications. Placement of IV catheters involves a small amount of damage to the vessel. The body can repair this damage by forming a clot. In some instances, an inappropriate amount of clotting occurs and the clot breaks off and forms an obstruction (thrombus) within the vessel lumen (Fig. 3.6). Thrombus formation is provoked by catheters that are rigid or have rough surfaces. In addition, some catheter materials allow seepage of certain components causing additional insult to the vessel. This is referred to as the reactivity of the catheter and is a feature that varies according to the materials used (Waddell 2004).

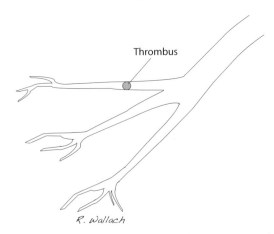

Figure 3.6. Thrombus formation in the vascular space is a complication associated with intravenous catheter placement. Illustration by Rachel Wallach.

Polyurethane

- Flexible material
- Can retain shape throughout longer dwell times
- Low reactivity
- Excellent choice for longer term catheters
- Fairly low risk of thrombosis

Teflon

- Rigid material
- Allows for easy insertion
- Leads to increased incidence of vessel damage
- Prone to kinking
- Higher incidence of thrombus formation than other materials
- Not suitable for long-term use

Silicon

- Extremely flexible
- Can make insertion difficult: guidewire required for placement
- Very low reactivity
- Excellent for long-term dwell

Polyvinyl Chloride and Polypropylene

- High reactivity
- Not widely available due to rate of complications

Three styles of IV catheters are generally seen in small animal practice: butterfly, over-the-needle, and through-the needle types.

Butterfly catheters

These devices use a short needle attached to a length of plastic tubing with a syringe-compatible port (Luer) on the distal end. Between the distal end of the needle and the tubing are wings used for directing the needle during placement (Fig. 3.7A).

The rigidity of the needle makes it an inappropriate choice for long-term fluid therapy. Movement of the cannula within the vessel can cause damage to vessel walls and lead to perivascular delivery of medication. Despite this fact, some clinical situations may require that the butterfly catheter be secured in place for a short duration (delivery of injectable anesthetic as a slow bolus). The wings can be used as anchors for tape to provide additional stability. This type of catheter can be used for a brief infusion, delivery of anesthetic, or collection of blood in most small animals. The sharpness of the needle improves ease of placement and increases patient comfort during venipuncture.

Butterfly catheters are available with a needle length of 1 to 3 cm and tubing length between 8 and 30 cm. Needles are available in sizes between 18 and 27 gauge.

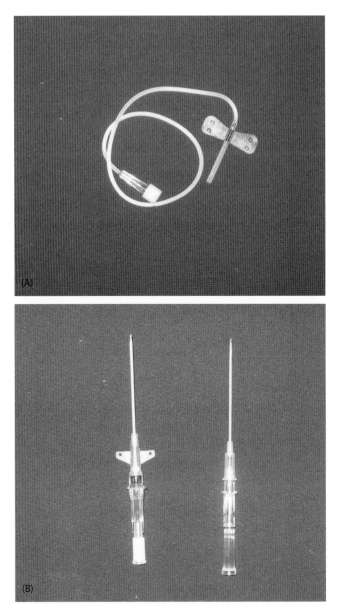

Figure 3.7. (A) Butterfly needles can be used for blood collection but are not appropriate for long-term delivery of intravenous fluids. (B) Over-the-needle catheters are preferred for intravenous catheterization.

Over-the-needle catheters

Over-the-needle catheters are composed of a metal stylet covered by a flexible cannula (Fig. 3.7B). The stylet has a bevel at the end and terminates with a sharp point. The exterior cannula, the catheter, has a slightly tapered end that is blunt.

The stylet guides the catheter through the skin and introduces it into the vessel (Fig. 3.8). The entire length of the stylet should not be advanced into the patient. The stylet is maintained in place until it is apparent the catheter is within the lumen of the vessel

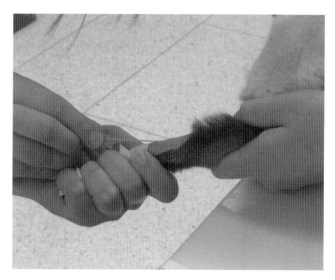

Figure 3.8.   Correct hand position for cephalic intravenous catheter placement.

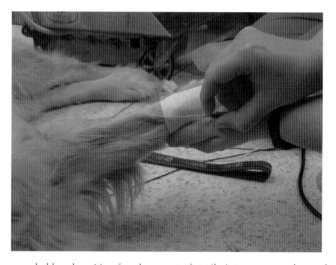

Figure 3.9.   Recommended hand position for placement of sterile intravenous catheter placement.

(Fig. 3.9). The catheter is advanced until the hub reaches the point of insertion (Fig. 3.10). The stylet is removed once the catheter is seated within the vessel.

One of the benefits of over-the-needle catheters is the similarity in size of catheter and stylet. Because the catheter slides over the outside of the stylet, the hole created by the stylet is no greater in diameter needed for introduction of the catheter. This minimizes leakage at the site of insertion.

This style of catheter is used with great frequency in veterinary medicine. It provides versatility with respect to the intended use of the catheter. Over-the-needle catheters can be used for fluid therapy, direct arterial blood pressure monitoring, serial arterial blood collection, and as a placement aid for central lines (modified Seldinger technique).

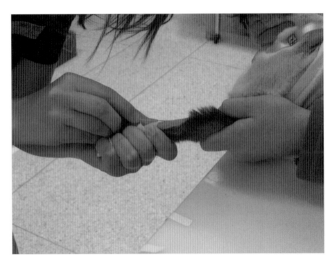

Figure 3.10. Index finger can be used to advance catheter off stylet.

Catheters can safely dwell at one site for several days providing they are patent and evaluated a minimum of once daily for any sign of redness or inflammation. Many practitioners schedule replacement of over-the-needle catheters every 72 hours. It has been demonstrated that catheters may remain in place for up to 7 days without complication (Mathews and Brooks 1996). Current trends suggest that increased dwell times are not necessarily the cause of complications or of increased incidence of infection (Marsh-Ng et al. 2007). Over-the-needle catheters may remain in place as long as they are functional and necessary and the patient has no sign of discomfort.

Some over-the-needle catheters are equipped with wings that lie on either side of the hub (at 0°and 180°). Critics of the over-the-needle catheter claim the catheter is difficult to secure. As a result the catheter moves in and out of the skin at the point of insertion and contaminates the venipuncture site by introducing bacteria found on the integument (Waddell 2004). This drawback is minimized, although not completely eliminated, by the existence of wings on the catheter hub. The wings can be used to secure the catheter onto the patient's limb using white medical tape. Securing the wings stops the catheter from rotating within the vessel and reduces the amount of movement in and out of the skin.

Over-the-needle catheters are typically used in peripheral vessels. Due to the anatomic features of most feline and canine patients, catheter location occasionally leads to obstruction of flow. If catheters are placed proximally on a limb, flexion of a joint often occludes the catheter. This is a minor drawback that can be avoided if appropriate attention is paid to catheter positioning at time of placement.

Nursing considerations

When placing these catheters care must be taken not to remove and replace the stylet within the lumen of the catheter. It is sometimes helpful to back the stylet out of the catheter and examine the catheter for evidence of blood flow that has not reached the distal end of the stylet. This is not good practice because reintroduction of the stylet causes microscopic injury to the tip of the catheter. In extreme cases the stylet may not reach the end of the catheter but rather puncture through the wall of the catheter while being reintroduced. Fraying or burring of the proximal end of the catheter causes damage to vessel walls, increasing the potential for development of thrombosis (Spencer 1982).

Securing over-the-needle catheters in place is an important step in preventing catheter-related complications. A simple method using four pieces of white medical tape has proven successful in the Ontario Veterinary College Teaching Hospital's small animal intensive care unit.

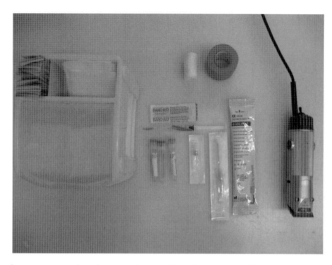

Figure 3.11. Supplies necessary for placement of sterile intravenous catheter.

Supplies (Fig. 3.11)

- Luer adapter (PRN Adapter by Becton Dickinson)
- Two pieces medical tape (~2 cm width) long enough to wrap around patient's limb
- Two pieces medical tape (~1 cm width) long enough to wrap around patient's limb
- One adhesive bandage with sterile cotton pad in middle (Band-Aid)
- Bandage material for padding (Conform by Kendall)
- Self-adhering bandage material (outer layer) (Vetrap by 3M)

Method (Fig. 3.12A–D)

- Thin tape adhesive side up placed under wings of catheter then folded back and wrapped around limb adhesive side down
- Thin tape, adhesive side down, anchor short end on wing using nondominant thumb, wrap under luer adapter and over second wing (makes shape of V) then around patient limb
- Gentle pressure is applied to V shaped tape to encourage catheter to sit toward patient
- Apply sterile adhesive bandage with catheter insertion site being covered only by sterile gauze square
- Avoid having adhesive tape covering point of insertion
- Apply first thick piece of tape over wings and around limb
- Apply second thick tape, adhesive side down in same manner as the second thin piece of tape

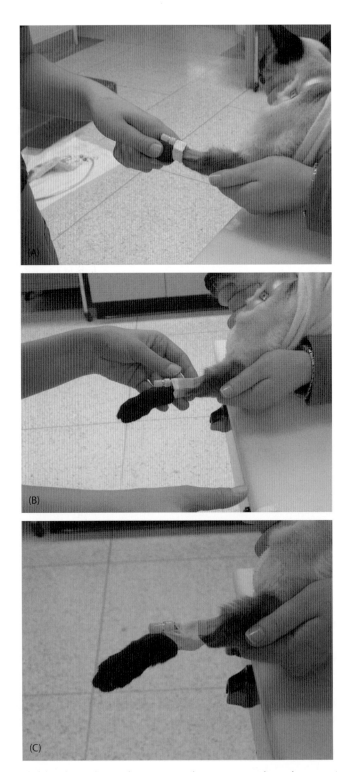

Figure 3.12. (A–D) The thumb can be used to exert gentle pressure on the catheter, maintaining it within the vessel, while the technician secures the appropriate pieces of tape. Strips of tape are used to secure the catheter to the patient's limb.

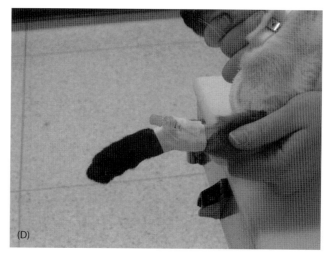

(D)

Figure 3.12. *(Continued)*

- Apply padding: start at distal limb and travel proximally (Figs. 3.13 and 3.14)
- For distal limbs, paw may be included but two toes should be visible and palpable
- Cover entire shaved area
- Apply self adhering outer bandage layer (Fig. 3.15)

Through-the-needle catheters

Through-the-needle catheters are long flexible catheters contained within a sterile plastic sheath before placement. The sheath is attached to the proximal end of the catheter at the base of the needle. Once the needle is placed the catheter is passed through the needle into the vessel (Fig. 3.16A–C)

Needle sizes range from 16 to 22 gauge and are between 3 and 5 cm in length. Catheters are available from approximately 20 cm to over 60 cm in length.

The entire through-the-needle system is closed, which helps maintain sterility during placement. Catheters can be placed into the jugular vein or through a medial or lateral saphenous vein. Insertion at any of these locations should place the end of the catheter within the cranial vena cava if the catheter is an appropriate length.

A surgical preparation of the chosen site is performed before placement. The needle is inserted through the skin. It is helpful to pick up a small section of skin and pass the needle through the tented skin and into the SC space before attempting insertion into the vessel. Once the needle has passed through the skin, the vessel is located and the needle punctures the vessel wall and enters the vessel lumen. A small flash of blood can be visualized in the proximal end of the catheter if needle placement is successful. At this point the catheter is advanced, using the outer sheath, until the entire catheter is seated within the vessel. The needle is withdrawn completely from the skin and enclosed within the needle guard or peeled away depending on the type of catheter used. The needle guard is secured to the patient and the catheter site is bandaged using a layer of padding and an outer adhesive layer. It is beneficial to use a lighter colored outer wrap

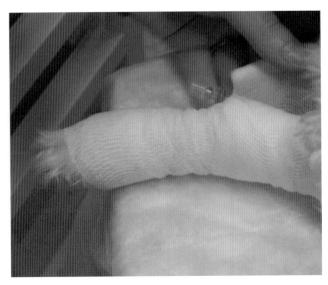

Figure 3.13. A layer of cotton gauze is used as a base layer of padding on the limb. Bandages should be placed from the toes in a proximal direction.

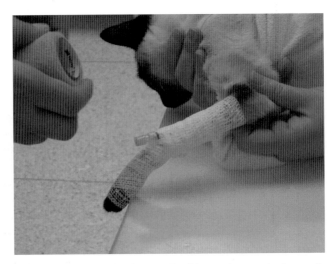

Figure 3.14. Padded layer of gauze. The technician should try to leave only the two longest toes visible at the distal end of the bandage (not the entire paw).

on jugular catheter bandages so any occurrence of strikethrough bleeding does not go unnoticed.

The catheter's position within the vena cava has many benefits. Measurement of central venous pressure is achieved via placement of a central line. Medications delivered through a central venous catheter achieve a higher concentration of drug in the blood vessels surrounding the heart (Drobatz 1999). This is particularly helpful during cardiopulmonary resuscitation.

The size of the vena cava and its associated volume of blood flow permit collection of blood samples with greater ease than via peripheral vessels. Sampling through a central line also facilitates collection of more substantial volumes. With a slightly faster draw time, blood drawn from a central line can be used for tests, such as a coagulation panel,

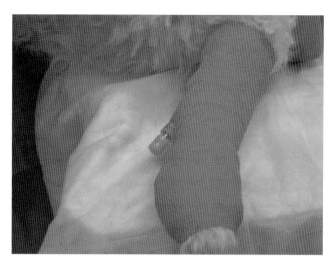

Figure 3.15. A layer of self-adhesive bandaging is used as an external layer.

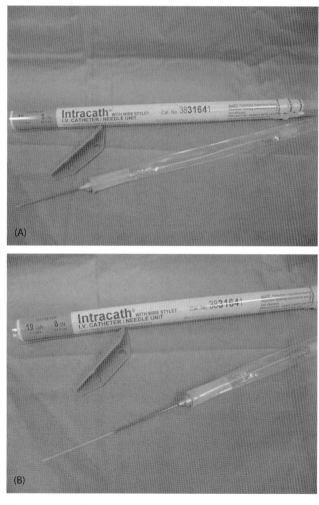

Figure 3.16. (A–C) Through-the-needle catheters may be used for central venous catheterization.

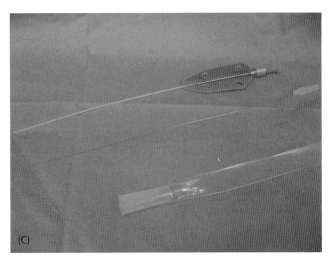

(C)

Figure 3.16. *(Continued)*

that are often not feasible when using a small peripheral vessel. An additional benefit of through the needle catheters is that blood collection is achieved without repeatedly invading the patient. This is a significant contribution to the overall comfort of the patient.

Repeated needle puncture of ports or luer adapters may compromise their integrity. Routine changes of fluid lines and luer adapters are good practice. Although catheters can remain in place indefinitely, lines and luer adapters should be changed every 72 hours. As an additional safety measure, ports may be swabbed with gauze square or cotton ball soaked in a bacteriostatic solution before any injection.

Samples may be drawn from the catheter using a three-syringe technique:

Materials

- One syringe with 3 mL heparinized saline (1 IU/mL)
- One syringe with 0.5 to 1.5 mL heparinized saline
- One syringe with no additives; appropriate size for sample needed
- Bacteriostatic swab for injection port
- Blood collection vials

Technique

- Pause fluid infusion and clamp line at point closest to patient but distal to injection port
- Swab port before introduction of each needle
- Using small heparinized saline syringe, inject approximately half the volume into the catheter being careful not to empty syringe
- Apply negative pressure to syringe and withdraw blood from catheter using slow steady pressure
- Mix blood with heparinized saline by gently inverting the syringe once or twice
- Recall that catheter is now full of fresh whole blood and can clot if too much time passes at this stage
- Remove blood sample using empty syringe and place sample in required vials

- Slowly inject heparinized blood sample into catheter ensuring there are no blood clots in syringe (blood should not be able to clot in heparinized syringe)
- Use 3 mL heparinized saline flush to clear catheter of any blood
- Use caution with volume of heparinized saline administered to patients receiving heparin therapy
- Remove only the volume of blood needed for analysis to avoid iatrogenic anemia

Through-the-needle catheters permit delivery of multiple types of fluids. Positioning within the vena cava allows for safe delivery of hyperosmolar fluids such as total or partial parenteral nutrition (Mazzaferro 2007).

As the name implies, IV placement of this type of catheter is achieved by advancing the catheter through a needle. To accommodate passage of the catheter, the inner diameter of the needle must be larger than the outer diameter of the catheter. This is a drawback associated with this style of catheter. The needle puncture creates a hole that is larger than the space occupied by the catheter once it is in place. Bleeding and leakage of fluids can occur at the insertion site (Spencer 1982).

Another potential difficulty encountered with through-the-needle catheters involves securing the needle and needle guard once the catheter is in place. Needle guards can be sutured and/ or glued to the patient's skin. In some instances, movement of skin in the cervical region alters the positioning of the needle guard and causes a kink in the catheter as it enters the SC space. Similar difficulties can arise with needle guards affixed to a distal hind limb. Patient movement may apply pressure to the needle guard and cause kinking at the point of insertion. This complication is not a concern with through-the-needle catheters placed via peel-away needles.

Multilumen Catheters

Double-, triple-, quadruple-, and five-lumen catheters are available for use as central venous catheters (Figs. 3.17 and 3.18). Double- and triple-lumen catheters are used frequently in intensive and critical care settings within veterinary medicine. Separate

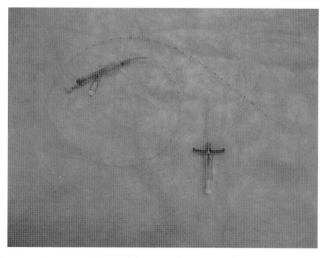

Figure 3.17. Peel-away catheters can be used for central venous catheterization.

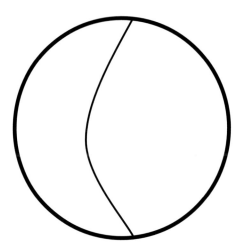

Figure 3.18. Double-lumen catheters are separated into two entirely separate compartments (lumens) within one catheter.

lumens permit simultaneous delivery of multiple fluid types as well as medications that are incompatible with other infusions. Total or parenteral nutrition can be delivered via one lumen while medication, crystalloid fluids, or other therapeutics are delivered safely, but separately, through the same catheter.

Multilumen catheters are appropriate for long-term use in patients whose peripheral access has been exhausted or in patients that require serial blood sampling.

Catheters are available in many sizes and lengths and can suit the largest canine patient to a small feline patient. Double-lumen catheters range from 4F to 14F in lengths of 5 to 7 cm. Triple-lumen catheters start at 5.5F and are available up to 12F depending on the manufacturer. These are available in lengths between 8 and 60 cm. Quad-lumen catheters start at 8.5F and are larger than what is necessary for most small animal patients.

Multilumen catheters are placed by the modified Seldinger technique. A minimum of two people are involved in this procedure. A second person is required even if the patient is anesthetized because the operator cannot simultaneously occlude the vein and place the catheter.

The entire procedure is performed with strict adherence to sterile technique (Figs. 19–29). A large margin is clipped and surgically prepared. The operator should remain sterile for the duration of the catheter placement. If the operator prefers to flush the multilumen catheter with heparinized saline before placement, this must also be done using sterile technique.

A small catheter or introducer needle is used to gain access to the vessel. Many of the central venous catheter kits provide an introducer needle; however, an 18- or 20-gauge over-the-needle peripheral catheter may be used in its place.

A guidewire or J wire is passed through the introducer and advanced several centimeters into the vessel. The needle is withdrawn and a vessel dilator is passed over the guidewire. A small incision is made in the skin at the point of insertion of the guidewire to facilitate introduction of the dilator. A moderate amount of force is needed to pass the dilator through the vessel wall. The dilator serves to widen the opening surrounding the guidewire so the larger diameter of the catheter can pass through. When the dilator is removed, sterile gauze may be applied at the point of insertion because bleeding often occurs. The catheter is fed onto the guidewire. It is important to maintain a hold on the guidewire while advancing the catheter. The guidewire will appear through the distal injection port. The operator must continue to hold the guidewire until the catheter is seated within the vessel and the guidewire can be removed.

A small amount of blood is aspirated from the catheter until the air that was in the catheter is collected into the syringe. The catheter can then be flushed with heparinized saline. The same procedure is repeated for each port. The catheter is then secured in place using suture and/or glue. Sterile gauze can be applied to the point of insertion and covered with an adhesive drape to seal out any contaminants. A layer of padding is applied over the adhesive drape and followed with an adhesive layer of bandage. Expandable adhesive bandage material that is light in color is a good choice for the outer wrap because it is soft, flexible, and light enough in color that any amount of strikethrough is readily apparent. The injection ports may be secured to the outer wrap

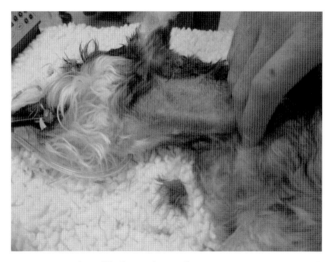

Figure 3.19. A generous area is shaved before catheter placement.

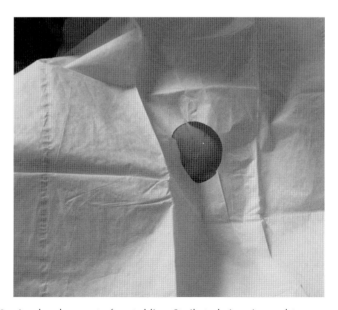

Figures 3.20–3.29. Jugular placement of central line. Sterile technique is mandatory.

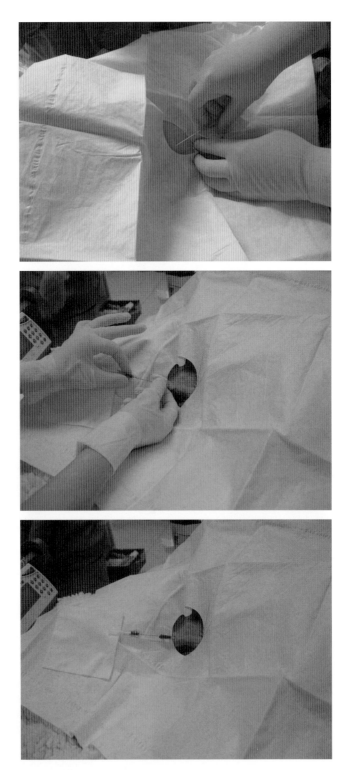

Figure 3.20–3.29. (*Continued*)

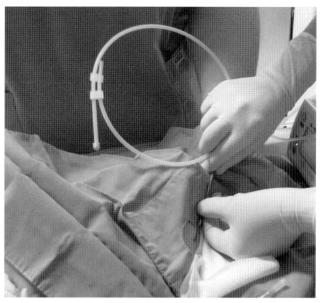

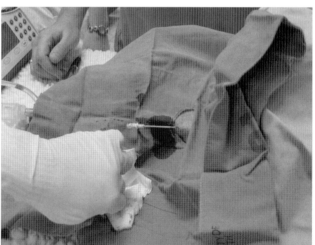

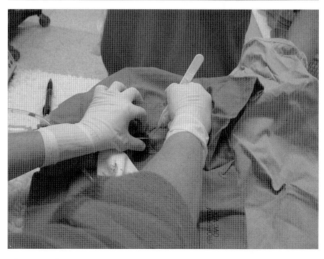

Figure 3.20–3.29. (*Continued*)

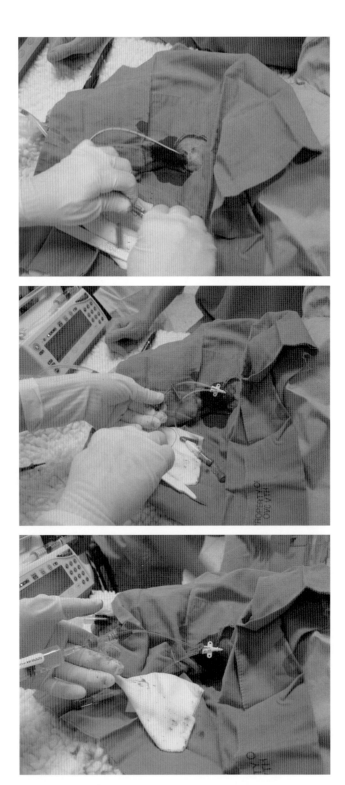

Figure 3.20–3.29. (Continued)

before connection to fluid lines. This will provide an additional anchor for the catheter and further decrease its chances of being accidentally dislodged.

 ## Nursing considerations

Patients undergoing placement of central lines (through the needle or modified Seldinger technique) should be sedated where cardiovascular status permits. This procedure requires technical expertise and is accomplished with greater haste if the patient is comfortable and still. Topical anesthetic such as lidocaine cream may be applied to the clipped area approximately 20 to 30 minutes before the procedure. This will provide additional comfort to the patient and facilitate placement of the introducer needle or over-the-needle catheter.

It is possible to advance the guidewire into the heart during placement of the multilumen catheter. If the guidewire enters the right atrium it may instigate arrhythmias. Monitoring heart rate and rhythm by means of an electrocardiogram can alert the operator to placement of the guidewire within the heart. If this occurs, the wire does not need to be removed entirely from the patient. It is likely that it only needs to be withdrawn by a few centimeters. Cardiac rhythm should return to normal once the guidewire is appropriately positioned within the proximal vena cava.

Through-the-needle and multilumen catheters can be used in many of the same situations. Each style of catheter requires a certain degree of technical expertise. If the personnel responsible for placement of the catheter have experience placing over-the-needle peripheral catheters, placement of central lines is a skill that can be quickly learned.

A study comparing catheter placement via the modified Seldinger technique with through-the-needle technique found that each method presented a similar level of challenge to an operator who had no previous experience with either. The most significant difference was that placement via the modified Seldinger technique took a longer time. Success rates were similar for each method. Further comparison found that blood collection took the same length of time from each catheter type (multilumen vs. through the needle) (Portillo et al. 2004).

With respect to vascular trauma, the modified Seldinger technique for placement of a central venous catheter caused less damage than the through-the-needle catheter when compared at postmortem. All of the through-the-needle catheters were found to have caused hematomas, whereas less than 90% of the modified Seldinger technique catheters resulted in the same findings. In addition, the average size of hematomas caused by the through-the-needle catheters was double that of the catheters placed by the modified Seldinger technique (Portillo et al. 2004).

Chapter Summary

Many routes are available for administration of fluid therapy. Selection should be made on a patient-by-patient basis, considering the signalment of the animal, the urgency of its needs, and the nature of its illness. The GI tract is an appropriate route for fluid therapy in patients that suffer no preexisting compromise of their digestive system. This route is appropriate for slow replacement of fluids and not suitable for patients in a hypovolemic crisis. The GI route is used via patient eating and drinking, via nasoesophageal feeding tube, or via esophagostomy or gastrostomy tube. Esophagostomy and gastrostomy tubes are reserved for patients requiring longer term therapy.

SC administration of fluids is convenient, economical, and technically available to most small animal practices. Its use is appropriate for treatment of mild dehydration. This route is not appropriate for critically ill patients due to the slow absorption of fluids from the SC tissue.

The intraperitoneal space can accommodate relatively large volumes of fluid. This route is not widely used in small animal practice due to the potential for serious complications. Redistribution of fluids is slow, which makes this route an inappropriate choice for hypovolemic or severely dehydrated patients.

IO delivery of fluids is underused in small animal practice. This route provides an alternative to IV therapy when illness has lead to cardiovascular collapse and subsequent difficulty obtaining venous access. Fluids delivered to the IO space are redistributed quickly, making this route an appropriate selection for hypovolemic patients. Technical ability and availability of appropriate materials may be limiting factors.

The IV route is an extremely versatile means by which fluid therapy is administered. This route provides access for delivery of crystalloids, colloids, blood products, and parenteral nutrition. Large volumes of fluids may be delivered into the vascular space, which is particularly important in severely compromised patients. IV catheters are available in a vast number of materials, gauges, and lengths.

IV therapy relies on appropriate selection and use of catheters. The three main types of catheters are butterfly catheters, over-the-needle catheters, and through-the-needle catheters. These are useful for short-term, moderate, and long-term use, respectively.

Guidewire catheters placed via the modified Seldinger technique are another style of catheter used in small animal patients. These catheters, along with most through-the-needle catheters, can be used in the jugular vein or through a peripheral vein to access the cranial or caudal vena cava, respectively. Catheters that terminate in this location are referred to as central venous catheters or central lines. They are frequently used for measurement of central venous pressures and collection of serial blood samples in intensive and critical care patients.

Review Questions

1. When is it inappropriate to use the enteral route for fluid therapy?
2. What is important regarding the length of the nasoesophageal (NE) tube that is selected for a given patient?
3. What are the landmarks used for measuring an NE tube?
4. What volume of fluid can safely be administered at each subcutaneous (SC) injection site?
5. Under which circumstances should the SC route not be selected for fluid therapy?
6. Name two significant advantages to the intraosseous (IO) fluid route.
7. Name two drawbacks of the IO route for fluid delivery.
8. Name four sites frequently used for IV access in cats or dogs.
9. With respect to safety and decreased incidence of catheter-associated complications, what catheter material is highly recommended for small animal patients?

Answers to the review questions can be found on page 222 in the Appendix. The review questions are also available for download on a companion website at www.wiley.com/go/donohoenursing.

Further Reading

Abrams-Ogg, A. 2003. Critical and supportive care in pediatrics. Proceedings of the Western Veterinary Conference.

Burrows, C. 1982. Inadequate skin preparation as a cause of intravenous catheter-related infection in the dog. *J Am Vet Med Assoc* 180:747–749.

DiBartola, S., and S. Bateman. 2006. Introduction to fluid therapy. In S. DiBartola, ed. *Fluid, Electrolyte, and Acid-Base Disorders in Small Animal Practice*, 325–343. St. Louis: Saunders.

Drobatz, K. 1999. Triage and initial assessment. In L. King and R. Hammond, eds. *Manual of Canine and Feline Emergency and Critical Care*, 1–6. Cheltenham, UK: BSAVA.

Gelens, H. 2003. Intraosseous fluid therapy. Proceedings of the Western Veterinary Conference.

Greene, C., and J. Hoskins. 1990. Drug and blood component therapy. In J. Hoskins, ed. *Veterinary Pediatrics*, 29–42. Philadelphia: Saunders.

Maki, D., and M. Ringer. 1991. Risk factors for infusion-related phlebitis with small peripheral venous catheters. *Ann Intern Med* 114:845–854.

Marsh-Ng, M., D. Burney, and J. Garcia. 2007. Surveillance of infections associated with intravenous catheters in dogs and cats in an ICU. *J Am Anim Hosp Assoc* 43:13–20.

Mathews, K. 2006. Monitoring fluid therapy and complications of fluid therapy. In S. DiBartola, ed. *Fluid, Electrolyte, and Acid-Base Disorders in Small Animal Practice*, 377–391. St. Louis: Saunders.

Mathews, K., and M. Brooks. 1996. A prospective study of intravenous catheter contamination. *J Vet Emerg Crit Care* 6:33–43.

Mazzaferro, E. 2007. Intravenous catheterization. *NAVC Clinician's Brief*, 37–40.

Mensack, S. 2008. Fluid therapy: options and rational administration. *Vet Clin Small Anim* 38:575–586.

Michell, A., R. Bywater, et al. 1989. Routes and techniques of fluid administration. In *Veterinary Fluid Therapy*, 121–148. Oxford, UK: Blackwell.

Olsen, D., B. Packer, et al. 2002. Evaluation of the bone injection gun as a method for intraosseous cannula placement for fluid therapy in adult dogs. *J Vet Surg* 31:533–540.

Portillo, E.M., A. Mackin, et al. 2004 Comparison of the modified Seldinger and through-the-needle jugular catheter placement techniques in the dog. *Proc Am Coll Vet Intern Med Conf.*

Spencer, K. 1982. Intravenous catheters. *Vet Clin North Am Small Anim Pract* 12:3 533–543.

Tan, R., A. Dart, and B. Dowling. 2003. Catheters: a review of the selection, utilization and complications of catheters for peripheral venous access. *Aust Vet J* 81:136–139.

Waddell, L.S. 2004. Advanced vascular access. Proceedings of Western Veterinary Conference.

Wingfield, W.E. 2002a. Emergency vascular access and intravenous catheterization. In W.E. Wingfield and M.R. Raffe, eds. *The Veterinary ICU Book*, 58–67. Jackson, WY: Teton NewMedia.

Wingfield, W.E. 2002b. Fluid and electrolyte therapy. In W.E. Wingfield and M. R. Raffe, eds. *The Veterinary ICU Book*, 166–188. Jackson, WY: Teton NewMedia.

Internet Resources

www.norfolkaccess.com/Catheters.html#Anchor-Catheter-49575.

Fluid Pumps and Tools of Administration

4

Administration Sets

Administration sets are the sterile lines used to deliver fluids to the patient. A spike that breaks the seal on the bag or bottle of fluids; a drip chamber; one or more clamps to halt flow; and one or more injection ports are found on standard administration sets. Additional features such as filters, Y-type ports, micro and macro drip specifications, and length of fluid lines can vary significantly.

The variety of features available with administration sets allows for patient-specific selection. The technician should consider the size of the patient, its health status, and potential fluid needs before selecting an administration set. This is of particular importance in patients whose fluids are not being delivered via infusion pump. Fluid infusion pumps facilitate delivery by allowing the volume of fluid required per hour to be programmed by the hospital personnel. This eliminates the need for manual calculation of drip rates and allows flexibility with respect to selection of drip chamber size.

Drip chambers

The drip chamber is a compartment that lies at the end of the fluid line closest to the fluid bag or bottle (Fig. 4.1). It is primed during the setup of the line and maintains a constant volume of fluid within the compartment until its source is depleted. The chamber is primed by gently squeezing its sides once or twice and allowing it to fill to a designated fill line approximately halfway up the wall of the compartment. Completely filling the drip chamber with fluid prevents the technician from evaluating the rate or quality of fluid flowing through the line. Maintaining the chamber at approximately

Fluid Therapy for Veterinary Technicians and Nurses, First Edition. Charlotte Donohoe.
© 2012 Charlotte Donohoe. Published 2012 by John Wiley & Sons, Inc.

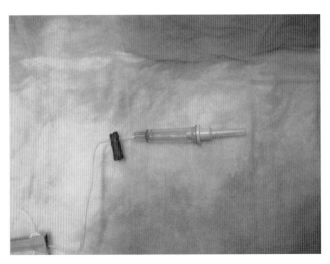

Figure 4.1. A drip chamber is attached to the bag of sterile intravenous fluids. Drops can be counted in this chamber to estimate flow rate and to ensure fluids are flowing properly.

half its capacity prevents large volumes of air from passing into the line and subsequently into the patient.

Drip chambers are available in different sizes. The sizes represent the number of drops delivered by the chamber per milliliter of fluid. Two sizes that are useful in small animal practice are 10 gtt/mL and 60 gtt/mL. It is easier to tailor the fluid rate using a 60 gtt/mL drip chamber for small canine and feline patients. The 10 gtt/mL set is referred to as a macro drip, and the 60 gtt/mL is referred to as a micro drip. Additional sizes are available for use in large animal patients.

Once the drip chamber is attached to the fluid source, it is important that the bottom of the chamber (attached to the fluid line) hangs below the fluid source. If the fluid line and drip chamber hang above the fluid source, the air that rises to the top of the chamber will flow into the line and eventually into the patient (Fig. 4.2).

Clamps

Most fluid lines have a series of plastic clamps that can occlude the flow of fluids at different levels throughout the line. Rolling clamps have a wheel that is advanced on the line and exerts increasing or decreasing pressure on the fluid line depending on the direction in which the wheel is rolled (Fig. 4.3). Flow can be completely obstructed using the rolling clamp. Patients receiving fluids without the advantage of an infusion pump have their rate of fluid delivery adjusted using this clamp. It is important to monitor the position of the clamp and the drip rate of the fluids at frequent intervals. If a pump is not responsible for delivering fluids, the rate can be inadvertently adjusted with accidental movement of the rolling clamp. It is possible to disrupt flow entirely or to deliver a fluid bolus, each of which could be dangerous for the patient.

Injection ports

Several injection ports lie within the line of the administration set (Fig. 4.4A, B). The ports can be used for injection of medication, catheter flushes, or for continuous rates

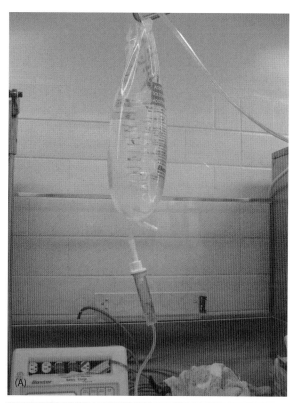

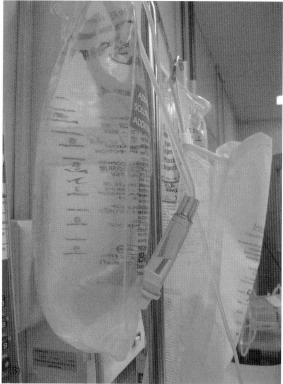

Figure 4.2. (A) Drip chambers must be suspended in this manner to avoid air flowing into delivery set. (B) Hanging the drip chamber in this position allows air and not fluid into delivery set.

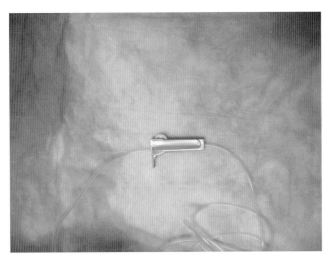

Figure 4.3. Roll clamps are included in lines to adjust flow rate.

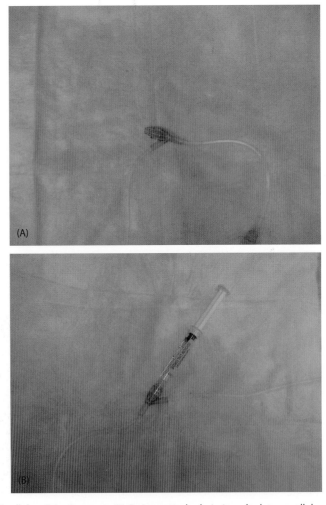

Figure 4.4 (A) Needleless injection port. (B) Syringe attached via Luer lock to needleless injection port.

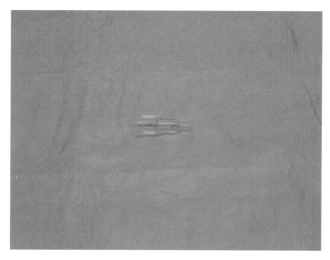

Figure 4.5. Needle-lock devices can be used to piggyback additional fluids (such as infusions of narcotic analgesics) into the main fluid line. These are used with needle-compatible infusion sets. A needle is seated in a plastic sheath that locks onto the fluid line once the needle is inserted into the port. Opposite end of sheath is the Luer port, attached to a syringe or to the catheter end of a fluid line. This device allows a connection between two lines or between a syringe and an infusion set that theoretically cannot come apart. With excessive patient movement, the needle-lock device may be disrupted or develop small leaks.

of infusion of medications piggybacked onto the main fluids. Extended or frequent use of injection ports can weaken the rubber and compromise the integrity of the port. Fluid infusion sets should be changed at least every 72 hours to maintain safety and sterility (Mathews and Brooks 1996).

Specific devices exist that facilitate one fluid line being connected to another via an injection port (piggybacking). The devices have a Luer on one end and a needle on the opposite side. The needle is contained within a sheath that locks onto the primary line. The Luer side (opposite the needle) is attached to a second infusion set. The fluid from the second infusion set passes through the needle into the lumen of the primary infusion and is delivered concurrently.

These devices are useful in practices that frequently have constant rates of infusions added on to primary fluid infusions. The ability to lock the secondary line onto the primary line is a major advantage (Fig. 4.5).

Where needle-locking adapters are not available, a hypodermic needle may be attached to a fluid line and piggybacked onto the primary line via the injection port. The main disadvantage to this setup is the ease with which the needle can accidentally slip out of the port.

At the Ontario Veterinary College Teaching Hospital, injection ports are wiped with 70% isopropyl alcohol before invasion with any type of needle or needleless system. Because small animal patients' fluid lines are occasionally in contact with the ground (during canine walks) or with the urine, vomit, or feces of a critically ill patient, wiping with an alcohol swab is a means of cleansing the injection port before use.

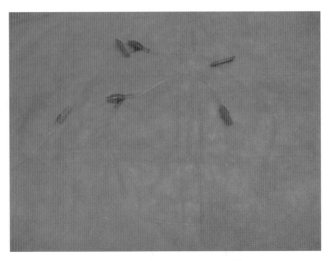

Figure 4.6.   Extension sets add length to delivery sets and provide additional injection ports.

Extension Sets

A single administration set is often not long enough to compensate for the movement of a patient within a kennel or a run. Fluid delivery sets with additional injection ports can be used to extend the length of the original drip set. Extension sets have Luer adapters on either end that are compatible with drip set and catheter, respectively. The extensions do not have a drip chamber and can be used in succession to increase the length of the fluid line (Fig. 4.6).

Extended fluid lines are beneficial and can contribute to the safety of the medical team in cases where a patient is fractious or defensive and unapproachable. Chemical restraint can be administered from a safe distance using one of the many injection ports on the fluid extension sets.

Burettes

A burette (trade name: Buretrol) is an instrument that can be used as a part of the fluid delivery set (Fig. 4.7). It is a plastic cylindrical chamber designed to hold smaller volumes of fluid. There is a vent on the top of the chamber as well as an injection port. The chamber has a volumetric scale on its side to allow for measurement of fluid. The burette has a universal spike on one end and a port that is compatible with a universal spike on the other end. The line between the fluid bag and the burette is equipped with a roll clamp. The line leaving the bottom of the burette is equipped with a straight clamp. Burettes are placed within the fluid line, between the fluid bag and the drip chamber.

A burette may be used to infuse a specific volume of fluids, a dose of medication over a set amount of time, or as a continuous rate infusion. Where infusion pumps are not available, the burette provides added safety by decreasing the likelihood that a patient receives a dangerously large volume of fluids. The line between the bag and the burette may be clamped to allow delivery of the small volume within the burette and nothing further from the fluid bag.

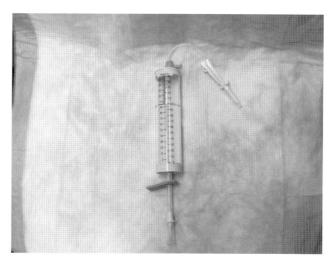

Figure 4.7. Burettes can be used to infuse medication over predetermined lengths of time.

Delivery of medications is achieved by fully or partially filling the chamber and adding the dose of medication into the fluids. In this manner, the fluids carry the dose of medication to the patient as a slow and steady infusion.

Example A

A patient is on a fluid rate of 75 mL/hr. The patient is scheduled to receive 400 mg of an intravenous (IV) medication as a slow push (over 20 minutes). The burette is filled to 25 mL with IV fluids and the 400 mg of medication is injected through the port at the top of the chamber. The fluid rate is continued at 75 mL/hr and the 25 mL of fluid containing the medication is infused over 20 minutes. Once the medication is delivered, the burette must be refilled promptly to avoid air passing into the delivery set.

Example B

A patient receiving fluids at 25 mL/h requires a constant rate infusion (CRI) of analgesics. The prescribed dose is 0.2 mg/kg per hour. If the animal is 10 kg, its dose is 2.0 mg/h. To make up an infusion that will last for 6 hours, the burette is filled to 150 mL (6 hours worth of fluids) and 12 mg of the analgesic medication is added. The concentration of the medication is 10 mg/mL, which means that 1.2 mL of analgesic is added to 149 mL of fluid. Note that 1 mL of fluid is removed to accommodate for the volume of medication being added. This will deliver a CRI of analgesics to the patient over a 6-hour period of time.

Miscellaneous Administration Sets

Vented sets

Specific administration sets are necessary for fluids being delivered from a plastic or glass bottle. If the container cannot collapse in response to the vacuum created by the siphoning fluids, the flow will cease. This is not of concern with traditional fluid bags

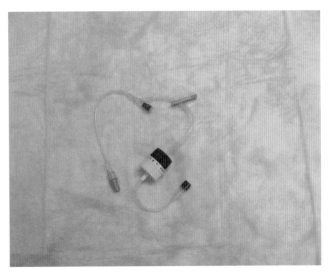

Figure 4.8. Flow regulator systems are used in administration sets for patients not on infusion pumps. These systems adjust fluid delivery rate and are calibrated in milliliters per hour.

because they can change their form in response to fluid volume. Vented administration sets may be used with fluid bottles to eliminate the accumulation of negative pressure within the bottle.

Rate flow regulator system

The rate flow regulator system is a section of infusion line equipped with a dial that sits within the line (Fig. 4.8). It is used to dial a specific number that corresponds with a flow rate for a given patient. These must be used with extreme caution in the busy critical care setting. Because the Dial-a-Flo infusion systems do not have any electrical component, there is no notification or alarm to alert the technician there is a problem with an infusion. Further, with mobile patients, it is not uncommon for lines to become tangled or kinked. The Dial-a-Flo system uses gravity rather than a positive pressure flow (such as with volumetric infusion pumps). If the line or catheter is less than perfectly positioned, it is possible that the gravitational flow of fluids will not overcome the minor obstruction.

An advantage to the flow regulator system is that the technician is not required to count drops to determine a rate of flow. In addition, by setting the flow regulator to a preselected rate, there is less opportunity for accidental overdose.

The rate prescribed by the clinician is selected on the dial and the designated volume should be delivered in milliliters per hour. Ranges vary, but most of these systems accommodate between 5 and 250 mL/h (Abbott Product Information).

Filters

Administration sets with inline filters must be used for delivery of blood products (Fig. 4.9). By removing larger particles from the blood product, the filters improve the safety of their IV administration. The filters remove white blood cells, fat, platelet

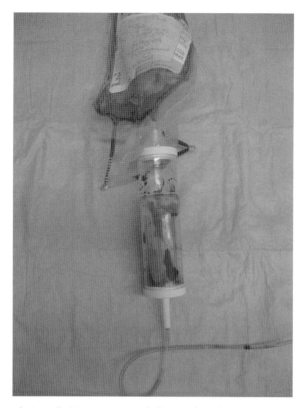

Figure 4.9.   Blood transfusion administration set with filter in drip chamber.

microaggregates, and blood clots that may have formed within the product (Mathews et al., 2006). Microaggregates are bundles of microscopic particles that can form in stored blood products. Most filters used in transfusion sets have pores that are 170 μm in diameter; other sizes are available.

Y-type infusion sets

As the name implies, these infusion sets are Y shaped and have two universal spikes, each with an inline filter, and are connected to a communal administration set. The main advantage to the Y-type sets is the ability to administer two products simultaneously. For example, if packed red blood cells and fresh frozen plasma are available from the same donor, the patient may receive concurrent infusions from each individual bag through the Y-type set.

Pressure bags

Pressure bags are used to increase the rate of flow of whichever type of fluid is being administered (Fig. 4-10). The pressure bag consists of opposing panels and two open ends. The length of the bag varies according to the size of the fluid bag it is meant to encase. Pressure bag sizes include 500 mL, 1, 3, and 5 L. The front panel is made of

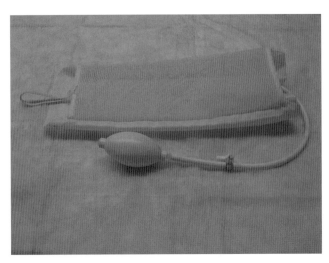

Figure 4.10.   Fluid bags are inserted into pressure bags. Pressure bags are pumped full of air, compress the fluid bag, and facilitate fast delivery of fluids.

mesh to facilitate observation of the fluid level within the fluid bag. The back panel is a double layer of fabric connected to a hand pump. The bag of fluids is placed within the pressure bag, and the pump is used to inflate the back panel. As the panel inflates, pressure increases and squeezes the fluid bag forcing fluid out through the drip chamber at an increased delivery rate. A pressure gauge on the bottom of the pressure bag indicates the amount of pressure being applied to the bag of fluids. There are also cautionary markings that indicate safe and unsafe inflation pressures.

Volumetric Infusion Pumps

Fluid infusion pumps are a standard of care in human hospitals (Fig. 4.11). The same is true of their presence in emergency and referral veterinary hospitals. Although infusion pumps are not as common in private practices, they are becoming more so.

An infusion pump is an excellent tool that facilitates and simplifies the administration of fluid therapy to veterinary patients. When used properly an infusion pump can save time, improve accuracy of dosing, and manage multiple infusions, thus allowing for more productive use of the technician's time.

Infusion pumps are made by many different manufacturers and are available in several different styles. Some are capable of managing one infusion (one fluid bag and one administration set); others are capable of managing three or four infusions at once (Fig. 4.12A, B).

Benefits of infusion pumps

Once a fluid type and delivery set has been selected for a patient, an infusion can be started quite quickly with the help of an infusion pump. If the animal's rate of fluid delivery has been decided ahead of time by the clinician, the rate and volume to be delivered are set on the pump and the infusion begins. Loading fluid lines into the pump

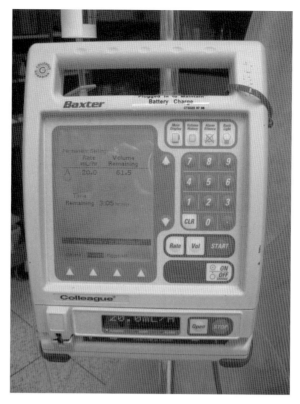

Figure 4.11. Infusion pumps come in many different styles. Single pumps are a popular choice in small animal practice.

is done with relative ease and becomes a simple and fast process once the veterinary technician has some amount of experience with the pump.

Volumetric infusion pumps deliver fluids with a high degree of accuracy. Additional precision is achieved through alarms that indicate when flow is not progressing at the rate at which it was prescribed. Infusions delivered *without* a pump may significantly slow or cease altogether if patient position or catheter patency prevents flow. Without an audible notification that the flow has changed, it may be difficult for the veterinary technician to promptly observe this change. Occlusion alarms on infusion pumps alert the technician to a change in flow rate, which allows the problem to be identified and corrected immediately. As such, the pumps contribute significantly to the accurate delivery of fluids.

Infusion pumps also notify the veterinary technician, via alarm, if a significant volume of air is in the fluid line. This notification allows the technician to remove the air from the line, preventing it from flowing into the patient. Fluids being delivered without the benefit of an infusion pump may silently carry small volumes of air through the delivery set and into the patient.

Drawbacks of infusion pumps

Perhaps the biggest drawback associated with infusion pumps is their cost. Despite the number of benefits associated with pumps, cost can be prohibitive.

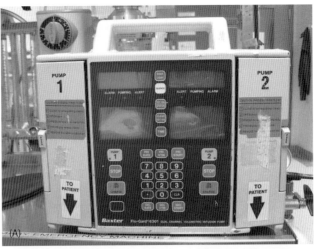

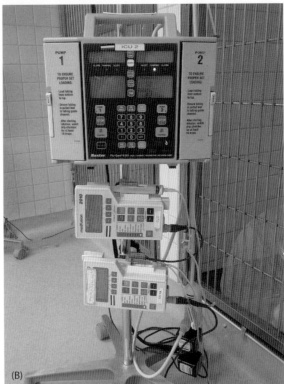

Figure 4.12.   (A) Double infusion pumps can be used for a single patient on multiple infusions or for two separate patients. Pumps should be clearly labeled. (B) Some critical care patients require multiple infusion pumps in addition to double pumps.

Some of the infusion pumps available for veterinary medicine can only be used with a specific infusion set. The infusion sets cannot typically be used with other pumps, and in some cases cannot be used without a pump. The need for such specific accessories increases the cost associated with use of the pump. There are many infusion pumps available that are designed for use with standard infusion sets, thus making use of equipment that already exists in the inventory of the average veterinary hospital. Before selecting an infusion pump for the veterinary hospital, it may be worthwhile for the technician to seek feedback from other fluid pump users. Peer comments and experience may highlight advantages and drawbacks associated with certain infusion pumps. This can contribute significantly useful information and potentially avoid the purchase of a notoriously frustrating or disappointing piece of equipment.

 ## Nursing considerations

There are features on most infusion pumps that are largely the responsibility of the technician. Although these are not consistently identified by the same title on all pumps, the features they represent are standard.

Rate

The rate is the speed with which the fluids are delivered to the patient. Measurement is made in milliliters per hour (mL/hr). This parameter is entered at the start of the infusion and is a variable prescribed by the veterinarian.

Fluid infusion pumps allow for expedient rate changes. By pausing the infusion, a new rate may be entered on the keypad, and delivery starts at the new rate as soon as the infusion is restarted.

Pumps can deliver fluids at extreme rates. Capacities differ between manufacturers, but it is not uncommon to be able to deliver rates as low as 0.5 mL/h or as high as 999 mL/h. The technician must exercise great care when programming the infusion rate.

Volume to be infused

The volume to be infused (VTBI) is another value set by the technician at the beginning of the infusion. This setting provides an end point for the pump. When this point is reached, an alarm sounds, notifying the health care team that the desired volume has been delivered to the patient. This is a useful tool because it provides a convenient point at which the patient can be reevaluated and the progress of fluid therapy assessed. It is important to resist the urge to program a large volume to be infused in an attempt to prolong the time between audible alarms. Instead, the VTBI should be revisited frequently, and each reprogramming should be for no greater than 2 hours at a time. For example:

■ Patient receiving 20 mL/h of fluids
■ VTBI set for 20 mL and patient is rechecked in 1 hour
■ Fluid therapy well tolerated
■ VTBI set for 40 mL and infusion continues for 2 hours
■ Patient is reevaluated; VTBI can continue to be set in 40-mL increments

Setting fluid boluses

It is vital that veterinary technicians understand the principles of rate and volume to be infused if they are responsible for setting infusion pumps to deliver fluid boluses.

Once the veterinarian has prescribed a bolus, technicians must be confident in their calculations and concepts. There are several ways to calculate rate and volume; the following is one example:

A 20-kg dog is prescribed a 10 mL/kg bolus to be delivered over 15 minutes. The volume of the bolus will be 10 mL/kg × 20 kg = 200 mL. Therefore the *volume to be infused* is 200 mL. To set a pump to deliver 200 mL over 15 minutes, the technician needs to determine what the rate must be in milliliters per hour. The following equation is helpful:

$$\text{Rate (mL/h)} = [60 \text{ min/h} \times \text{volume to be infused (mL)}]/\text{infusion time (min)}$$

For the preceding example, the equation would be:

$$\text{Rate (mL/h)} = (60 \text{ min/h} \times 200 \text{ mL})/15 \text{ min}$$

$$\text{Rate (mL/h)} = 12,000/15 = 800 \text{ mL/h}$$

The infusion pump would be set with a rate of 800 mL/hour and a volume of 200 mL to be infused. This would give the patient a 10 mL/kg bolus over 15 minutes. Confusing the rate with the volume to be infused can be catastrophic. In our example, the patient would receive a volume of 800 mL instead of 200 mL.

It is good practice to verify calculations and/or check them with a coworker before setting infusion pumps because it increases the safety of the infusion.

Total volume

This feature calculates a current total of the volume of fluid that has been infused since the beginning of the infusion. It is not programmed by the technician, but she or he must clear the previous totals before starting each new patient's infusion. Failure to do so allows volume to accumulate from one patient to another in some brands of pumps. It is advisable that the veterinary technician become familiar with whichever style of pump is in use to clarify whether this feature automatically resets with each new infusion.

Silence

The silence button is a feature used with great frequency in high-volume hospitals. Any alarm that sounds can be temporarily muted by depressing the silence button. Technicians find this key particularly useful because it can become taxing if several pumps are alarming simultaneously. The silence feature will be in effect for a predetermined amount of time before it allows the alarm to return to its alert sequence.

Lock

The lock feature is typically located at the back of the infusion pump. It is often a switch that protrudes from the pump slightly so that accidental activation of the switch is improbable. Once the lock feature is activated, changes cannot be made to any of the infusion settings. In essence, the keypad is rendered useless while the lock is on. (This can be frustrating when the alarm is triggered because the silence button is also disabled by the lock).

At the Ontario Veterinary College Teaching Hospital, the intensive care unit technicians frequently use the lock feature when a specific volume or temporary infusion is being administered. A crystalloid bolus, 30-minute infusion of medication, or a blood transfusion can be initiated by the technician and then the pump can be locked. The number of technicians, clinicians, and students who could inadvertently reset the volume to be infused without realizing the volume *should not* have been reset is quite high. By locking the pump, the technician forces the subsequent operator to reconsider which course of action is appropriate once the alarm sounds.

Troubleshooting volumetric infusion pumps

As with any equipment used in the veterinary hospital setting, technicians must develop a repertoire of solutions for a variety of difficulties they may encounter.

Placement of fluid line

Careful placement of the fluid line is essential to avoid fluid traveling in an inappropriate direction. Each infusion pump has a single specific method to load the infusion set, and directions must be followed without exception. If the line is put into the pump backward, the motion of the pump will reverse the flow, and in extreme cases, blood will flow from the animal into the line.

Air

Infusion pumps are designed to notify the health care team if a large volume of air should pass through the line in the pump. When this situation arises, the infusion stops to avoid air going into the patient's vasculature. When removing the air from the line the technician must practice sterile technique. The fluid line is clamped at the closest point to the patient. Heparinized saline flush (1 unit heparin per milliliter of saline) is administered into the injection port, proximal to the clamp, and into the catheter to maintain patency. The door to the pump must be opened and the line removed from the pump. The injection port is swabbed with an antibacterial solution. A 6-mL or 12-mL syringe and 20-gauge needle can be used to evacuate the air from the injection port closest to the air, but the port should be between the air and the patient. Fluid from the bag will be evacuated with the air, but the patient will be unaffected because the line has been clamped and is closed to the patient.

   Once the air has been removed from the line, the syringe and needle are discarded appropriately. The line is replaced in the pump and the door is closed. The line can be unclamped once it has been replaced and locked into the pump. The pump is restarted and should flow without alarms if the air has been effectively removed.

Occlusions

The occlusion alarm is one of the more frequently heard alarms. Volumetric infusion pumps have sensors that detect if pressure is rising within the section of fluid line within the pump. Any compromise to the rate of flow will cause a subsequent increase in the inline pressure and trigger the occlusion alarm. Factors that impede flow are numerous and in some cases unavoidable.

   Administration sets that have been in use for 2–3 days occasionally develop kinks or crimps where they have repeatedly been positioned within the pump mechanism. These interruptions often lead to an occlusion alarm. Placing a new section of the administration set within the pump mechanism can alleviate this problem. However, if the administration set is beginning to show its wear, it is likely that the set should be completely changed for a new one.

It is possible to catch the administration set in the door as it is being closed. This is not often immediately apparent but may be the source of the occlusion alarm and should be investigated.

Veterinary patients are often responsible for occluding their own lines and triggering occlusion alarms. Animals that circle or pace in their kennels can cause such severe twists in their lines that fluid can no longer flow. In many instances, this is unavoidable. The line may be clamped at the port most proximal to the patient. A heparinized saline flush will maintain catheter patency while the line is untangled. In addition, clamping the port proximal to the patient ensures that when the fluid line is removed from the pump and untangled, there will be no sudden flow of fluids into the patient.

Occlusions may also arise due to catheter-associated problems. IV catheters that have been improperly secured, have shifted due to tremendous patient movement, or have become clotted will prevent smooth progression of flow. In addition, catheters that have caused vascular trauma, inflammation, or thrombophlebitis will impede flow and cause an occlusion alarm. Catheters should be investigated as a cause for any occlusion alarm if there is no other obvious culprit. Changes in catheter patency can be subtle and difficult to recognize because the catheters are not easily visible to the technician due to bandaging. Daily evaluation of the catheter site is necessary, but more frequent inspection might be warranted if fluid infusion becomes problematic.

High rates of infusion, such as with fluid boluses, can be subjected to a greater number of occlusion alarms. Because the fluid rate is higher than normal, a slight obstruction or decrease in patency will cause a much faster buildup of pressure in the fluid line. In this instance, if the fluid rate can be safely decreased, even slightly, it may alleviate the occlusion pressure alarm situation. If it is not possible to decrease the rate of flow, a pressure bag may be the next best substitute to provide a high rate of flow without constant interruptions by pump alarms.

Syringe Pumps (Syringe Drivers)

A syringe pump is a tool with many uses in fluid therapy (Fig. 4.13). The pump is designed to infuse small volumes of fluid at rates that are generally slower than those achieved by volumetric infusion pumps. As such, a syringe pump may be used to infuse small volumes of fluid to a small patient during fluid therapy, finite volumes of blood products for transfusion medicine, continuous rates of infusion of narcotic analgesics, or singular slow infusions of medication.

There are many ways to deliver fluids using a syringe pump. It is helpful that the technician can program doses to be delivered by volume, by rate, by time, and by dose.

Several pieces of information must be entered into the syringe pump's processor to ensure accurate delivery of fluid. Syringe volume, syringe manufacturer, patient weight, prescribed dose, drug concentration, and infusion rate are the main variables programmed by the technician with each use of the syringe pump.

The syringe drivers are designed to accommodate a number of different syringe sizes; most are compatible with 1-mL to 60-mL syringes. Once the syringe has been loaded into the pump, it is necessary to indicate the syringe manufacturer. This is necessary because syringe shapes are not consistent throughout suppliers (Fig. 4.14).

After programming the brand of syringe and confirming that the pump has recognized the correct volume of syringe, the technician is responsible for programming the patient's

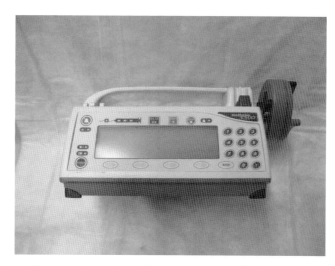

Figure 4.13. Syringe drivers can be used to deliver constant rates of infusions of medications or for single doses that are delivered over shorter periods of time.

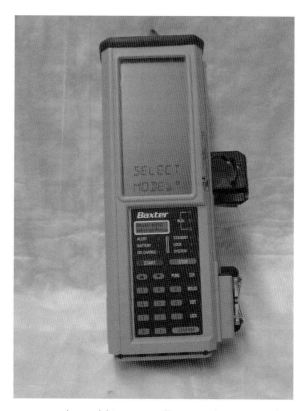

Figure 4.14. Syringe pumps are also useful in very small patients that require infusions at very low rates.

body weight, dose, and drug concentration (if needed for medication delivery) to complete the pump setup. If a single volume of fluids is being delivered, the technician can program a rate of flow and have the appropriate volume of medication drawn up in the syringe before setting up the pump. Setting up the syringe pump can be as simple or as complex as needed based on the type of infusion the patient is receiving.

Alarms

Syringe pumps are equipped with occlusion alarms, end-of-infusion alerts, and syringe-depleted notifications. In addition, these pumps are equipped with an alarm to indicate if the position of the syringe's barrel or plunger has been changed, rendering it nonfunctional.

The reasons a syringe pump occlusion alarm may sound are similar to those found with larger infusion pumps. Any impediment to the flow of fluids causes a fluid backup, an increase in volume, and subsequently pressure within the line. When the alarm is appreciated, the technician should appraise the patency of fluid lines and assess catheter site and catheter limb.

Troubleshooting syringe pumps

Syringe pumps are quite reliable and typically run with few complications. However, the complications that can and do arise can impart severe consequences if not handled appropriately. It is important to remember that despite the reliability of mechanical equipment used for fluid therapy, the use of this equipment can never entirely excuse technicians from using their skills of observation. Fluid bags and syringes should be assessed frequently to ensure that the volume expected to have been infused *has* been infused. Further, connections between fluid lines, needle lock adapters, and miscellaneous infusion lines should be monitored for any signs of wear or leakage.

Assessment of syringe pump function is often instigated by the sound of an occlusion alarm. The technician must respond promptly to the alarm and determine its cause. It has been demonstrated that alleviating an occlusion alarm can deliver a bolus (of the substance being infused) to the patient (Donmez et al., 2005). The size of the bolus varies depending on the size of syringe being used. The larger the syringe, the larger the bolus that the patient accidentally receives when the occlusion is alleviated. One study found that a 10-mL syringe led to a 0.09-mL bolus, and a 60-mL syringe led to a 1.03-mL bolus (Kim and Steward, 1999). In many cases, the delivery of a bolus of fluids at this volume would be inconsequential. However, if the syringe pump is being used for the delivery of medication, such as narcotics, inotropic, or antiarrhythmic drugs, delivery of this size of bolus could be detrimental to the patient. This danger is heightened if the patient is a neonate, small feline, or teacup canine breed.

It is unlikely that occlusions will be avoided in every infusion delivered to veterinary patients via syringe pump. To increase the safety of the infusion, the technician may choose to disconnect a section of the fluid line so that the potential bolus is not delivered to the patient. In addition, to decrease the size of an inadvertent bolus, the technician may choose to use a small-volume syringe for the infusion if possible to do so.

There are further benefits to using a small-volume syringe with a syringe pump. In addition to the decrease in size of inadvertent bolus previously mentioned, using a smaller syringe also contributes to increased promptness of the occlusion alarm (Kim and Steward 1999). Larger syringes led to an increased length of time between the onset of the occlusion and the sounding of the occlusion alarm. Smaller syringes had the opposite effect. In one study 7.4 minutes elapsed between onset of occlusion and onset of alarm when a 10-mL syringe was used. The same study found a delay of 84 minutes between occlusion and alarm when a 60-mL syringe was used (Kim and Steward 1999). These findings do not indicate that larger syringes should not be used with syringe pumps, but rather that the infusion must be continuously monitored to verify it is progressing according to plan.

Flow rate is another factor that contributes to the length of time between onset of occlusion and onset of alarm. Lower flow rates correspond with greater lag time between occlusion and alarm, whereas higher flow rates are associated with quicker onset of alarm (Donmez et al., 2005). If one considers that occlusion alarms respond to pressure elevations within the fluid line, it fits that higher rates would be quicker to increase inline fluid pressure. Because syringe pumps are primarily used for small infusions with relatively low flow rates, it behooves the technician to assess the line frequently to ensure forward flow.

Some syringe pumps are equipped with a function that allows the operator to program different levels of tolerance for inline pressure. It is safer to select a low pressure limit and tolerate higher sensitivity and more frequent alarms than to select a high tolerance for pressure and allow prolonged lengths of time to elapse before onset of the alarm (Hee and Lim 2002).

Chapter Summary

Infusion or administration sets are fluid lines that facilitate deliver of fluids to veterinary patients. These sets are composed of a universal spike, a drip chamber, multiple clamps, multiple injection ports, and a Luer adapter.

Drip chambers allow the technician to monitor the continuous fall of drops during infusion. In systems that do not involve a fluid pump, the drip chamber is used to count drops of fluid to verify flow rates. For this reason, the drip chamber must not be overfilled during priming. There is a fill line indicator on the chamber that demonstrates the fluid level that accommodates drip counting. The common sizes of drip chambers in small animal medicine are 10 and 60 gtt/second.

Miscellaneous adapters may be used in conjunction with the administration set to lengthen the fluid line, accept other infusions, filter blood and blood products, or infuse multiple fluid types simultaneously.

Burettes measure smaller volumes of fluid and have a gradation on the side of the chamber to facilitate measurement of volume. They are a helpful tool during emergency situations because they can house a small volume of fluids that is not dangerous to the patient should it be infused in its entirety. On the contrary, if fluids are started at the onset of an emergency, it is possible to focus on other immediate concerns and accidentally infuse a dangerous volume of fluids to the unstable patient if there is no burette in the fluid line. Further, burettes can be used to deliver constant rates of infusion of medications and/or analgesics over a predetermined amount of time. They are a precious tool in the critical care setting.

Volumetric infusion pumps are accurate and reliable and can be used with a large margin of safety provided the operator is well versed in management of the pump. Rate and volume to be infused are the primary features programmed by the technician at the beginning of the infusion. As the infusion progresses, it is the responsibility of the technician to maintain safe operation of the fluid pump and ensure that the volume to be infused is reached but not exceeded.

Syringe pumps are excellent tools that facilitate delivery of extremely small volumes of fluid via very low fluid rates. Smaller syringes are safer to use with syringe pumps than larger syringes.

The technician is responsible for setting a number of parameters to facilitate smooth infusion of drug or fluid. Occlusion alarms are often preset at a specific pressure point, but in some models, this feature can be programmed.

Occlusion alarms are triggered by a number of different issues. Alarms may be slow to sound if the fluid rate is low or the syringe size is large. Technicians must check IV lines and catheter sites frequently to ensure there are no problems with the infusion.

There are few negative aspects to using volumetric infusion pumps in the veterinary setting. Provided the technician is aware of the potential complications and can respond to alarms in a timely and effective manner, infusion pumps are an asset to any veterinary practice. Within the critical care setting, they are an indispensable tool.

Review Questions

1. Why should the drip chamber be positioned with the fluid line facing down?
2. Which drip chamber sizes are most frequently encountered in small animal medicine?
3. When is an inline filter a required characteristic of an IV administration set?
4. A variety of different syringe sizes can be used with syringe pumps. With respect to obstruction of flow, is it safer to use larger volume or smaller volume syringes?
5. List two benefits associated with burettes.

Answers to the review questions can be found on pages 222–223 in the Appendix. The review questions are also available for download on a companion website at www.wiley.com/go/donohoenursing.

Suggested Reading

Donmez, A., C. Araz, and Z. Kayhan. 2005. Syringe pumps take too long to give occlusion alarm. *Paediatr Anaesth* 15:293–296.

Hee, H., and S. Lim. 2002. Infusion technology: a cause for alarm. *Paediatr Anaesth* 12:780–785.

Kim, D., and D. Steward. 1999. The effect of syringe size on the performance of an infusion pump. *Paediatr Anaesth* 9:335–337.

O'Kelly, S., and J. Edwards. 1992. A comparison of the performance of two types of infusion device. *Anaesthesia* 47:1070–1072.

Mathews, K., and M. Brooks. 1996. A prospective study of intravenous catheter contamination. *J Vet Emerg Crit Care* 6:33–43.

Mathews, K., H. Scott, and A. Abrams-Ogg. 2006. Transfusion of blood products. In K. Mathews, ed. *Veterinary Emergency and Critical Care Manual*, 667–681. Guelph, Ontario, Canada: LifeLearn.

Metheny, N. 1992. Intravenous therapy. In N. Metheny, ed. *Fluid and Electrolyte Balance*, 149–168. Philadelphia: JB Lippincott.

Calculating Rates of Administration

5

Technical Calculations

The International System of Units is a classification of measurements used throughout the world. When referring to measurements made within this system, it is common to use the term *SI units*. The SI system includes terminology used to quantify scientific measures such as length, weight, electricity, and amount of substance. Table 5.1 lists the terms of particular interest in the study of fluid therapy.

Calculating the volume of fluid to be delivered to a patient and the rate at which it is to be delivered are the most fundamental calculations the veterinary technician must make. These values are prescribed, in part, by the veterinarian. It is the responsibility of the technician to calculate, initiate, and monitor the infusion to the patient and ensure that the prescribed fluid therapy is delivered without incident.

The fluid therapy prescription is arrived at through consideration of the patient's age, weight, hydration status, cardiovascular status, and health history. The clinician can determine the volume and speed with which fluids are delivered in several ways. In some cases, a calculation is made that takes into consideration the estimated percentage of dehydration, the volume lost, and the ongoing losses the patient is experiencing.

It is also common for the clinician to request that fluids be given at maintenance rate or a multiple of maintenance rate. This rate is based on the estimation that healthy adult cats and dogs lose approximately 50 mL/kg per day of fluids through the natural processes involved in metabolism (Mathews 1996). Metabolic water is lost in feces, urine, and through respiration. As such, the intravenous (IV) fluid required to replace these losses (when patients cannot do so for themselves) is deemed the *maintenance fluid rate* because it is designed to replenish naturally occurring losses.

Fluid Therapy for Veterinary Technicians and Nurses, First Edition. Charlotte Donohoe.
© 2012 Charlotte Donohoe. Published 2012 by John Wiley & Sons, Inc.

Table 5.1   SI Units Commonly used in Fluid Therapy

Name of Unit	Abbreviation	What It Measures
Meter	m	Length
Kilogram	kg	Weight
Second	s	Time
Mole	mol	Amount of substance

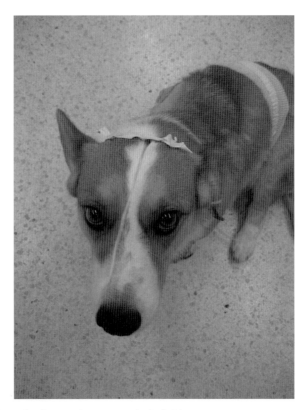

Figure 5.1. A healthy 15-kg dog requires preanesthetic fluids.

Calculating a maintenance rate

When the technician is given orders to start a patient on maintenance fluids, it is necessary to know the patient's weight and the rate accepted as maintenance for the given patient in a given hospital. For the purpose of this text, the previously mentioned rate of 50 mL/kg per day (or maintenance fluid rate) is used. Note that patient age and size play a role in determining maintenance fluid rates. Very young animals have a higher fluid requirement than middle-aged adult animals. This is due to the fact that in good health, 75%–80% of the total body weight of a puppy or a kitten is water. In contrast, the body water content of an adult animal is closer to 60% of their total body weight.

Size of the patient should also be considered when deciding on a maintenance fluid rate. Smaller animals actually have a higher maintenance fluid requirement than larger animals. For example, the maintenance fluid rate for a 6-kg patient might be 54 mL/kg per day, whereas the maintenance fluid rate for a 70-kg patient is more likely to be 29 mL/kg per day (Mathews 2006).

Example 1

A 15-kg dog is admitted to the hospital for a routine procedure (Fig. 5-1). The veterinarian requests that the dog receive Plasma-Lyte A (PLA) at the maintenance rate for 4 hours before the procedure.

- Maintenance is 50 mL/kg per day
- Body weight is 15 kg
- Rate = 50 mL/kg × 15 kg/24 hours
    - Units of kilograms cancel each other out
- Rate = 750 mL/24 h
- Rate = 31.25 mL/h
- Rate = 31 mL/h

If the clinician has prescribed that this rate be given for exactly 4 hours and no longer, the technician can then calculate the total volume the patient should receive.

- Total volume to be infused (VTBI) = 31 mL/h × 4 hours
    - Units of hour cancel each other out
- Total volume to be infused = 124 mL

The technician must consider other variables depending on the system used for the infusion. For example, if the infusion is being delivered via volumetric infusion pump, there are two settings to be programmed. Using the previous calculations, it is known that the rate is 31 mL/h and the VTBI is 124 mL. A fluid bag can be hung with no other adapters, and the pump will deliver the predetermined volume of fluids.

Another alternative is to hang a burette in the infusion line and fill it with 124 mL of fluid. This is not a necessary step but rather a course of action that increases the safety of the infusion. If another member of the patient care team were to continue the infusion once the pump had delivered the preprogrammed volume, the empty burette in the infusion line would encourage the person to investigate whether or not the delivery *should* continue.

Delivering the infusion without the benefit of a fluid pump would require further calculations. Once the rate is determined, it is necessary to set the drip rate for the infusion set. The technician proceeds through the steps required to determine the number of drops per second (gtt/s) required for a rate of 31 mL/h.

To calculate the drip rate, the technician must know the number of drops that the set delivers per milliliter. This information is available on the outside packaging of the drip set. For the purpose of this text, we assume a 15 gtt/mL set is in use.

- It is known from previous calculations that the patient requires 31 mL/h
- Determine the volume of fluid required per minute by dividing the hourly rate by 60 (there are 60 minutes in 1 hour)

- 31 mL/h/60 = 0.52 mL/min
- Another option is to multiply 31 mL/h × 1 h/60 min if it is easier to visualize the units that cancel out
- Once the rate per minute is known, it can be multiplied by the drip factor obtained from the packaging to determine the number of drops per minute
- 0.52 mL/min × 15 gtt/mL = 7.8 gtt/min
- It follows that 7.8 gtt/min × 1 min/60 s yields the number of drops per second that the patient should receive
- 7.8 gtt/min × 1 min/60 s = 0.13 gtt/s

Because counting 0.13 gtt is virtually impossible, the technician must work in units of time slightly greater than 1 second. By multiplying the preceding by a factor of 10, it is determined that 1.3 gtt are delivered in 10 seconds. Another calculation also yields a more user-friendly format. Once the number of drops per minute has been calculated, the equation can be reversed as follows:

- 60 s/7.8 gtt/min = 7.69 s/gtt
- One drop is delivered every 8 seconds by rounding up to the next whole number

It is easiest to count the number of seconds between drops for most infusions delivered to small animals.

A formula that makes the preceding calculations flow more smoothly is the following:

$$\text{Drops/min} = \text{total volume to deliver (mL)} \times \text{number of drops/mL} \div$$
$$\text{total time of infusion (min) (Metheny 1992)}$$

Using the data from the previous example, 31 mL × 15 gtt/mL ÷ 60 min = 7.76 gtt/min, approximately 8 gtt/min is a reasonable rate to watch and set up with a drip set. The 1-minute time frame could be further divided into more manageable segments if the technician so chooses. By dividing both sides of the rate by 4, it is determined that in a 15-second interval, the patient should receive roughly 2 drops of fluid.

Example 2

A 4-year-old male castrated domestic shorthair cat is presented to the hospital with a 48-hour history of vomiting and inappetence (Fig. 5.2). The cat weighs 3.8 kg. The clinician requests that the patient be started on fluids at two times the maintenance rate (often referred to as "twice maintenance").

- Fluid rate = maintenance rate × patient weight × 2
- Rate = 50 mL/kg per day × 3.8 kg × 2
- Rate = 380 mL/d
- Rate = 380 mL/d × 1 d/24 h
- Rate = 15.8 mL/h
- Next determine the rate in mL/min: 15.8 mL/h × 1 h/60 min = 0.26 mL/min
- Factor in the drip set 0.26 mL/min × 15 gtt/mL = 3.9 gtt/min
- To determine how many seconds between drops: 60 s/1 min × 1 min/3.9 gtt = 1 gtt/15.4 s

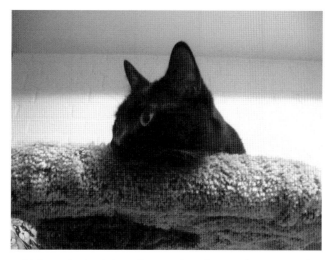

Figure 5.2. A 4-year-old domestic shorthair cat has a 48-hour history of vomiting and inappetence.

Administering 1 drop every 15 seconds is not ideal because this slow drip rate could allow a clot to develop in the catheter between drops of fluid. This example highlights one of the reasons that drip chambers are available in different drip factors. If the preceding example were calculated using a 60 gtt/mL drip chamber, one would anticipate that the drops would flow more frequently.

- Recall that it was calculated the patient needed 15.8 mL/h
- 15.8 mL/h × 1 h/60 min = 0.26 mL/min
- 0.26 mL/min × 60 gtt/mL = 15.6 gtt/min
- 60/15.6 gtt/min = 1 gtt/3.85 s; rounded up to 1 gtt/4 s

This is a more reasonable rate of flow in terms of maintaining catheter patency. As the preceding example illustrates, it is helpful to use a drip chamber with a greater number of drops per milliliter for smaller patients (i.e., <10 kg).

Example 3

A 32-kg, 6-year-old female spayed German shepherd presents to the hospital with a complaint of severe diarrhea, depression, and anorexia (Fig. 5.3). She is estimated to be 6% dehydrated. The clinician recommends that the dog be hospitalized and started on IV fluids. What is her fluid requirement over the first 24 hours of her hospital stay? Assume that a 15 gtt/mL drip set is being used.

- If the dog is 6% dehydrated, this estimation can be used to calculate an approximate volume of fluid that needs to be replaced.
- 6% dehydration = 6/100 × 32 kg = 1.92 kg
  - 1000 mL or 1 L of water weighs 1 kg; 1.92 kg = 1.92 L
- So at 6% dehydration, the 32-kg German shepherd is at a deficit of approximately 1.9 L
- Maintenance fluid requirements for the shepherd are calculated to be 50 mL/kg per day × 32 kg = 1600 mL/24 h

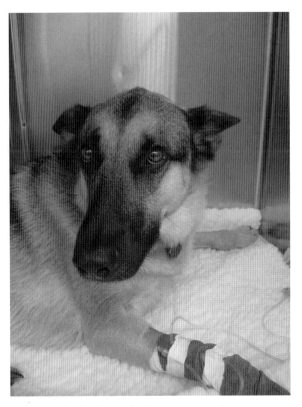

Figure 5.3. A 6-year-old German shepherd with diarrhea and depression.

The clinician requests that the dog's fluid deficit be replaced over a 24-hour period. The technician must calculate the volume of fluid needed to compensate for the patient's maintenance requirements in addition to the fluid deficit and replace the total of the two over 24 hours.

- Maintenance requirement 1600 mL + deficit 1900 mL = 3500 mL over 24 hours
- To deliver 3500 mL over 24 hours, the following calculations are made:
- 3500 mL/24 h = 145.8 mL/h (round up to 146 mL/h)
- 146 mL/h × 1 h/60 min = 2.43 mL/min
- 2.43 mL/min × 15 gtt/mL = 36.45 gtt/min
- 60 s/36.45 gtt/min = 1 gtt/1.6 s

If a volumetric pump was being used for this infusion, the rate would be set at 146 mL/h and the VTBI would be set to deliver 2- to 4-hour increments at this rate, 292 mL—584 mL at a time. The total volume that needs to be delivered in the 24-hour period is 3500 mL. Using a burette in the infusion line may be helpful for administration of medications for this patient, but the hourly fluid rate is almost equal to the volume of a burette. Refilling the burette every hour may not flow smoothly with the other activities taking place in the clinic and may prove to be an inefficient use of technician time.

The use of a rate flow regulator in the delivery set is also appropriate for this dog. The technician must evaluate the flow frequently and ensure that the bag is

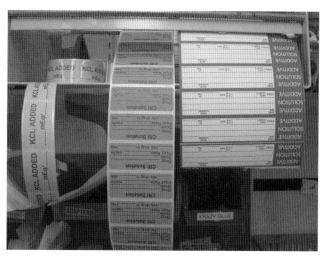

Figure 5.4. Additive labels should be used on all fluid bags to clarify what has been added, when it was added, and by whom.

emptying at an appropriate rate. It is often helpful to use a strip of white tape on a fluid bag to monitor the progress of fluids into the patient. Fluid level within the bag can be marked on the white tape in intervals, and the time can be recorded with the level marked.

Fluid additives

Patients receiving long-term fluid therapy often require supplementation of certain electrolytes to their fluid therapy regime (Fig. 5.4). Potassium chloride (KCl) is frequently used as a supplement in the emergency and critical care setting because many of the patients in this setting are hypokalemic as a result of their illness and subsequent lack of appetite. Solutions such as potassium chloride, potassium phosphate, and magnesium sulphate may be added to fluid bags to restore electrolyte balance to small animal patients. LRS and Normosol R are popular fluid choices for many patients on short-term fluid therapy. Note that these fluids do not contain a sufficient amount of KCl to maintain adequate levels for patients in ill health. KCl must be added to these fluids to supplement or support the patient's potassium level.

To calculate the appropriate volume for supplementation, it is necessary to know the concentration of the additive in use as well as the prescribed dose. Electrolytes may be added to full or partial fluid bags. For this reason, the technician must be able to calculate appropriate volumes rather that memorize the dose that is to be added to a full bag.

The clinician prescribes the rate of electrolyte supplementation. This prescription is typically in the form of a required concentration prepared in the primary fluid infusion. A hypokalemic patient might be prescribed KCl supplementation at a dose of 30 mEq/L. If the technician is starting the infusion and has an entire 1-L bag of fluids, the addition of 30 mEq of KCl is fairly straightforward. Once the concentration of KCl is known, it is used to determine the volume, in milliliters, of KCl to be added.

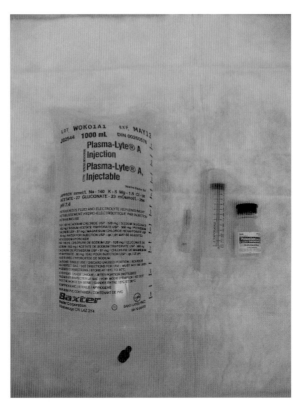

Figure 5.5. Potassium chloride is often added to intravenous fluids to supplement hypokalemic patients.

Example 1

Make up a 1-L bag of PLA with 30 mEq KCl/L (Fig. 5.5). A bottle of KCl is available in a concentration of 20 mEq/10 mL or 2 mEq/mL. It is necessary to find out what volume will supply 30 mEq of KCl.

- This is easily determined by cross multiplying and solving for x
- 2 mEq/1 mL = 30 mEq/x mL
- 2 mEq × x mL = 30 mEq × 1 mL
- 2x = 30
- x = 30 ÷ 2
- x = 15

To add 30 mEq of KCl to a liter of fluids, the technician must add 15 mL of KCl at the previously mentioned concentration.

Example 2

A severely hypokalemic patient is prescribed an infusion of 0.5 mEq/kg per hour of KCl for 4 hours. The patient is receiving PLA at a rate of 20 mL/h. The KCl infusion will be delivered via burette. The patient weighs 10 kg. The stock solution of KCl is provided as 20 mEq in a 10-mL bottle (2 mEq/mL).

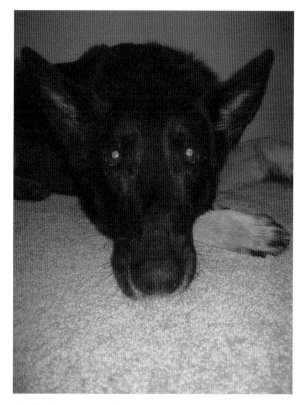

Figure 5.6. A German shepherd presents to the hospital and is found to be hypoglycemic on initial blood work.

- dose: 0.5 mEq × 10 kg/1 h = 5 mEq/h
- 5 mEq/h ÷ 2 mEq/mL = 2.5 mL/h of KCl
- 4 hours worth of this infusion would require 10 mL of KCl (4 × 2.5)

If the patient is receiving 20 mL/h of fluids, the 4-hour infusion will have a total volume of 80 mL (20 × 4). We know that of this 4-hour infusion volume, 10 mL must be KCl. To infuse the volume over the allotted time, it is preferable to combine 70 mL of PLA with 10 mL KCl for a total of 80 mL and a 4-hour total infusion time.

Example 3

A 45-kg German shepherd has presented to the hospital in a hypoglycemic crisis (Fig. 5.6). The dog has had two IV boluses of dextrose as well as 2 10 mL/kg boluses of PLA. The dog is now slightly more stable, and the clinician has requested that the patient's fluids be supplemented with dextrose. The prescribed fluid regime is PLA plus 5% dextrose as a constant rate infusion. The stock solution of dextrose is 50%. There is a burette in the administration set whose volume is 150 mL. The clinician requests that the burette be used initially; the bag can be supplemented once the patient's initial response to the infusion is documented.

To determine concentrations of solution the following equation is useful:

$$\textbf{Volume to add (mL)} = \textbf{strength required} \div \textbf{strength available} \times \textbf{final volume}$$

$$\text{-volume to add (mL)} = 5\% \div 50\% \times 150 \text{ mL (burette)} = 15 \text{ mL}$$

The following is another equation that is useful for calculating the volume of fluid to add to a solution to arrive at a desired concentration:

$$C_1 \times V_1 = C_2 \times V_2$$

For the previous example: $50\% \times V_1 = 5\% \times 150\,\text{mL}$

$0.5 \ V_1 = 0.05 \times 150$
$0.5 \ V_1 = 7.5$
$7.5 \div 0.5 = V_1$
$V_1 = 15 \text{ m}$

Both equations yield the same result. The technician has the liberty of choosing whichever equation he or she prefers.

Because 15 mL is being added to a 150-mL burette, it is preferable to remove 15 mL PLA from the burette before adding the dextrose.

Constant rates of infusion

In the emergency and critical care setting it is frequently necessary to deliver drugs to patients as a continuous infusion. This is achieved through administration via syringe pump, as an additive to a burette, or as an additive to a fluid bag. The drug is delivered at the same rate over a predetermined time period or within a predetermined volume of fluid.

Several pieces of information are required before the technician can make the necessary calculations and set up a constant rate of infusion (CRI). The infusion is prescribed as a dose per kilogram per minute, hour, or day. The dose can come in several different formats; milligrams and micrograms are the most common in the small animal setting. It is necessary to know the concentration of the drug and the weight of the patient. Depending on the method of delivery, it may be necessary to know the fluid rate as well.

Once the clinician has prescribed a CRI, the technician must calculate the dose with respect to the patient's weight. Further, if the infusion is going to be delivered in a fluid infusion, it is necessary to calculate how much drug is to be added to the fluid within the bag or burette.

Example 1

A 15-kg patient is prescribed a constant rate of infusion of butorphanol as an analgesic for some mild discomfort. The dose is 0.2 mg/kg per hour. The concentration of the butorphanol on hand is 10 mg/mL. The animal is currently on two times maintenance rate of fluids. There is a burette in the administration set.

■ Calculate the dose: 0.2 mg/kg per hour × 15 kg = 3 mg/h
■ The concentration of butorphanol is 10 mg/mL
　■ it is necessary to determine how many milliliters contain 3 mg

■ 3 mg/x = 10 mg/1 mL
■ Solve for x by cross multiplying: 10x = 3
■ x = 10/3
■ x = 0.3 mL
■ 0.3 mL of butorphanol will deliver 3 mg so the dose just calculated can be changed to 0.3 mL/h
■ If a syringe pump is available, the drug is drawn up in a syringe, the pump is programmed to deliver 0.3 mL/h, and the line is piggybacked into the main infusion line.
■ If the technician opts to deliver the drug in a burette, it is necessary to calculate a convenient volume of fluids to which the drug can be added.
■ The fluid rate for this patient is twice maintenance:

$$\text{Maintenance} = 50 \text{ mL/kg per day} \times 15 \text{ kg} = 750 \text{ mL/d}$$

$$2 \times \text{maintenance} = 1500 \text{ mL/d} = 62.5 \text{ mL/h (round to 63 mL/h)}$$

Most burettes can hold 150 mL; if the fluid rate is 63 mL/h, then filling the burette with 126 mL of fluid will provide enough for 2 hours of infusion.

■ Two hours worth of butorphanol can be added to the 2 hours worth of fluid in the burette, so it is delivered as a constant rate infusion.
■ It is vital that the burette be labeled according to the volume of additives it contains
■ 0.6 mL butorphanol in 126 mL fluid will provide the appropriate dose of analgesics for this patient
■ The drawback to this method is that the burette must be replenished every 2 hours.

This CRI could also be prepared in a bag of fluids, assuming that the infusion is going to continue for a prolonged amount of time.

■ The bag of fluids contains 1000 mL
■ At a rate of 63 mL/h, the bag should last for 15.9 hours:
   ■ 1000 mL: x hours = 63 mL:1 hour
   ■ x = 1000/63 = 15.9 hours
■ If the patient is receiving 0.3 mL/h of butorphanol, then multiplying this by the number of hours, the bag will last will yield the volume of butorphanol to be added to the bag.
   ■ 15.9 hours × 0.3 mL/h = 4.77 mL
■ The technician must add 4.77 mL of butorphanol to the bag of fluid to provide a CRI of butorphanol to this patient for the next 15.9 hours.
■ It is imperative that the bag be appropriately labeled with the volume and type of drug added.

Nursing considerations

When preparing medications for CRI, the technician must be familiar with the characteristics of the drug. For example, some drugs are light sensitive and must be protected once they have been removed from their original bottle. This is of particular interest when discussing CRIs because long infusions may expose drugs to light for prolonged periods of time. In the previous example, the butorphanol would have been exposed to light for nearly 16 hours. The technician must investigate whether or not it is safe to do so before setting up the infusion.

If it is likely that the patient's fluid rate will change throughout the duration of the infusion, it may not be practical to prepare an entire fluid bag with the additive to be delivered. As the fluid rate changes, the CRI is no longer delivered at the volume at which it was intended. The concentration in the bag is constant, so any change to fluid rate will drastically change the volume of drug being delivered.

- In example 1, 1000 mL of fluid contained 4.77 mL (47.7 mg) of butorphanol, which is equal to 0.0477 mg butorphanol/1 mL of fluid
- At twice maintenance the patient was getting 63 mL × 0.0477 mg = 3.005 mg/h of butorphanol.
- If the fluid rate is changed to 2.5 times maintenance the patient will receive 78.13 mL × 0.0477 mg = 3.72 mg/h of butorphanol, which exceeds the dose originally prescribed.

Changing fluid rates can significantly alter the dose of drug delivered to a patient. This is an important consideration for the technician when choosing the means of CRI administration.

Example 2

A 7-kg cat is recovering from a pelvic fracture repair. The cat is prescribed a CRI of fentanyl as an analgesic at a dose of 3 μg/kg per hour. The concentration of fentanyl is 50 μg/mL. The cat is receiving 22 mL/h of PLA.

- 3 μg/kg per hour × 7 kg = 21 μg/h
- 21 μg/h ÷ 50 μg/mL = 0.42 mL/h
- A full burette (150 mL) would last this cat for 6.8 hours at 22 mL/h
- 6.8 hr at 0.42 mL/h of fentanyl would require the addition of 2.9 mL of fentanyl.

Example 3

A 35-kg dog is prescribed a CRI of metoclopramide at a rate of 1 mg/kg per day. The concentration of metoclopramide is 5 mg/mL. How much metoclopramide does the dog need added to its fluid bag if the drip rate is 145 mL/h?

- Calculate the dose: 1 mg/kg per day × 35 kg = 35 mg/d
- Calculate the dose per hour: 35 mg/d ÷ 24 hours = 1.46 mg/h
- Calculate the volume per hour: 1.46 mg/h ÷ 5 mg/mL = 0.29 mL/h

The dog requires 0.29 mL/h of metoclopramide.

- Calculate how many hours of therapy are provided by one 1000-mL bag of fluids
- 1000 ÷ 145 = 6.9 hr/bag
- 6.9 hours of fluid × 0.29 mL/h of metoclopramide = 2.00 mL of metoclopramide to be added to the fluid bag

Table 5.2 Useful Conversions and Equations

Goal	Method	Example
Calculate % of solution	Weight in grams ÷ volume in milliliters × 100	1 g cephalexin ÷ 10 mL × 100 = 10%
Calculate concentration if % solution known	Move decimal to right one space and add a zero	5% dextrose = 50 mg/mL
Volume required to dilute to specific concentration	Strength required ÷ strength available × final volume	10% dextrose solution ÷ 50% dextrose solution × 1000 mL = 200 mL into 1-L bag of fluids
Determine volume required to obtain specific concentration	$C_1V_1 = C_2V_2$ C = concentration V = volume	How much 50% dextrose is added to 150-mL burette to make a 5% solution? $5 \times 150 = 50 \times V_2$ $V_2 = 15$ mL
Convert pounds → kilograms	Multiply by factor 0.45	2 l b × 0.45 = 0.9 kg
Convert inches → millimeters	Multiply by factor of 25.4	1 in × 25.4 = 25.4 mm
Convert fluid ounces → milliliters	Multiply by factor of 28.4	4 oz × 28.4 = 113.6 mL
Convert mL → liters	Divide by 1000	10 mL/1000 = 0.01 L
Convert liters → milliliters	Multiply by 1000	1 L × 1000 = 1000 mL

Nursing considerations

When adding very small volumes of drug to large volumes of fluid, it is uncommon to remove the volume of fluid that corresponds to the additive before its addition. However, if a large volume of drug is added into a volume of fluid, it is more accurate to remove an equal amount of the fluid before addition of the drug. For example, if the technician is preparing a 1-L bag of PLA as a 5% dextrose infusion, 100 mL of dextrose must be added to the bag. To maintain and improve accuracy, 100 mL of Plasmalyte should be removed from the bag before addition of the dextrose.

When preparing CRIs using very small volumes of additive, it is acceptable to add the drug to the fluid without removing an equal volume of fluid beforehand.

Example 3

A 33-kg Doberman is being treated for heart failure attributed to dilated cardiomyopathy. The clinician has prescribed dobutamine as a constant rate infusion at 5 µg/kg per minute. Dobutamine has been made up as a 0.5 mg/mL concentration in 0.9% sodium chloride. Calculate the volume of fluid to be delivered to the Doberman.

- Dose: 5 µg/kg/min × 33 kg = 165 µg/min
- Dose in milligrams: 165 µg/min ÷ 1000 µg/1 mg = 0.165 mg/min
- Calculate milligrams per hour: 0.165 mg/min × 60 min/h = 9.9 mg/h
- Calculate milligrams per hour: 9.9 mg/h ÷ 0.5 mg/mL = 19.8 mL/h
- The patient will receive 19.8 mL/h of the dobutamine solution in 0.9% NaCl.

Despite the technician's capability to calculate and convert figures, some facts inevitably must be committed to memory. Table 5.2 summarizes helpful fluid therapy conversions and equations.

Chapter Summary

This chapter summarized the veterinary technician's most frequent calculations. Perhaps the most basic calculation is the determination of fluid rate. This is prescribed by the clinician but may be calculated by the technician. The prescription may come in the form of milliliters per kilogram per day, or as a shorter form, it may refer to how many times maintenance the patient should be receiving. Once the rate of fluid delivery has been determined, it may be necessary to determine a total volume to be delivered over a set period of time. On an infusion pump, this is classically referred to as *volume to be infused*.

When an infusion pump is not available, the technician must calculate the fluid rate and then determine the number of drops per second (gtt/sec) that the patient requires to receive said fluid rate. In small patients it is more useful to calculate the number of seconds per drop because the former would require counting drops in fractions, which is not very accurate.

Once a patient's weight is known, it is possible to calculate the volume associated with an estimated percentage of dehydration. The percentage is converted into a fraction and multiplied by the patient's weight. The volume in liters is the patient's volume deficit. Clinician's orders may vary with respect to how slowly or how quickly this deficit is to be replaced. The maintenance rate of fluids must also be considered when calculating the rate of replacement.

Supplementing fluid therapy with electrolytes, dextrose, narcotics, and medications is a common occurrence in emergency and critical care settings. It is imperative that all calculations correspond to the correct body weight of the patient, the correct drug dosage, and the correct concentration of drug to be added. These two common equations can be used for this type of calculation:

1. $C_1 \times V_1 = C_2 \times V_2$
2. **Volume to add = strength required ÷ strength available × final volume**

Constant rates of infusion (CRIs) are another style of medication delivery commonly used in the critical care setting. CRIs can be used for efficient delivery of pain medication as well as to deliver medications that have a short duration of action. CRIs are calculated based on the concentration of the drug and the weight of the patient. They are prescribed in many different ways, with drug dose and units of time fluctuating depending on which drug is being administered.

When adding large volumes of medication or alternative supplement to a fluid solution, it is necessary to remove an equal volume of the solution before adding the medication. This is required to maintain the same final volume and ensure the drug will be delivered at the appropriate strength over the appropriate amount of time.

As with any calculation involved in daily practice, it is prudent that the technician always double-checks the math or have a coworker complete the same calculations for verification. It is far easier to correct a mathematical mistake before fluids or medications are administered to the patient than it is to deal with the repercussions of the same mistake after the fact. Errors in dosages are easily avoided by taking a few extra seconds to check calculations.

Practice problems

1. A hypoglycemic patient requires an infusion of 10% dextrose. The stock solution is 50% dextrose. Calculate the volume of dextrose to add to a 500-mL fluid bag.
2. A 25-kg dog is prescribed a continuous rate infusion of metoclopramide (5 mg/mL) at a dose of 2 mg/kg per 24 hours. The dog's fluid rate will be 100 mL/h. What volume of metoclopramide must be added to a 1-L bag for this patient?
3. A cat is admitted to the hospital after being hit by a car. Once the cat has been stabilized, received analgesics, and been fully examined, she is placed in a kennel. The cat is prescribed a CRI of butorphanol at 0.2 mg/kg per hour. The cat weighs 5 kg, and her fluid rate is 15 mL/h. Calculate the volume of butorphanol to be added to a burette that contains 75 mL of fluid.
4. A 12-kg diabetic ketoacidotic canine patient requires supplementation with potassium and phosphorus. The clinician would like to accomplish this by administration of KCl and potassium phosphate (KPO_4). The prescribed dose of KPO_4 is 0.02 mmol/kg per hour. The prescribed supplementation of potassium is 30 mEq/L. The patient has a new 1-L bag of fluid with no additives hanging and has a 150-mL burette in the administration set. Because the fluid therapy prescription is likely to change frequently, it is prudent to make up the current supplements for addition to the burette. The fluid rate is 50 mL/h. The concentration of KCl is 20 mEq per 10-mL bottle. The concentration of KPO_4 is 3 mmol phosphate/mL and 4.4 mEq potassium/mL. What is the volume of each solution that must be added to the patient's fluids to meet the requirements of the fluid prescription?
5. You are providing care to a patient that has just undergone a thoracic limb amputation. The analgesic plan for this patient is concurrent CRIs of fentanyl and ketamine. The dog weighs 43 kg. Her fluid rate is 130 mL/h. Her analgesics are prescribed as 3 μg/kg per hour of fentanyl and 0.2 mg/kg per hour of ketamine. Fentanyl is available with a concentration of 50 μg/mL and ketamine 100 mg/mL. Hint: With such a high fluid rate, it is practical to make up this infusion in a 1-L fluid bag.
6a. A 4-kg 6-year-old domestic shorthair cat is admitted to the hospital after being diagnosed with pancreatitis. The cat is prescribed a CRI of butorphanol, which is to be preceded by a loading dose of 0.2 mg/kg. The CRI will run at 0.2 mg/kg per hour. Initially, the cat is placed on 15 mL/h of PLA. There is a 150-mL burette in the line. The concentration of butorphanol is 10 mg/mL. Calculate the volume of butorphanol to be added to a full burette.
6b. After running the infusion for 5 hours, the clinician requests that the fluid rate be changed to 8 mL/h. How much butorphanol should be added to the remaining 75 mL of fluid?
6c. An alternate situation might be that the cat is very comfortable and the clinician asks that the CRI be decreased to 0.1 mg/kg per hour after the infusion has been running for 6 hours. What is a simple approach to adjusting the burette?
7. A hypotensive patient is prescribed a constant rate infusion of dopamine at 6 μg/kg per minute. The patient weighs 12 kg. Dopamine is supplied as a 5-mL vial with a concentration of 40 mg/mL.

7a. The orders are to make up a bag of dopamine for infusion using the contents of the 5-mL vial and combining them with a 250-mL bag of 0.9% NaCl. What is the concentration of the dopamine infusion in the bag in milligrams per milliliter?

7b. What is the concentration of the dopamine infusion in micrograms per milliliter?

7c. Calculate the infusion rate in milliliters per hour for the patient just described.

8. A hypotensive tachycardic patient is admitted to the hospital with a 4-day history of vomiting and anorexia. The current weight of the patient is 15 kg. The clinician orders a 15 mL/kg bolus over 15 minutes. At what fluid rate should the pump be set? What is the volume to be infused?

9. A 12-kg dog is admitted to the hospital and found to be 8% dehydrated. The clinician requests that the dog be started on fluids immediately and that the dog's fluid deficit be replaced over 24 hours in addition to its maintenance fluid requirements (50 mL/kg per 24 hours). Once the dog has IV access, the clinician also requests delivery of a 10 mL/kg bolus over 15 minutes.

9a. Calculate the rate and volume to be infused for the fluid bolus assuming that an infusion pump is being used. The maximum rate for infusion on the pump is 1999 mL/h.

9b. Calculate the dog's fluid rate for the first 24 hours of hospitalization.

Answers to practice problems

1. Concentration required/concentration available x volume required = volume to add
   - Volume of dextrose to add = 10%/50% × 500 = **100 mL of 50% dextrose is added to bag**
   - Can also be written as 0.1/0.5 × 500 = **100 mL of 50% dextrose**
   - Prior to addition of dextrose, 100 mL should be removed from bag to maintain same final volume.

2. Calculate rate with respect to patient's weight: 25 kg × 2 mg/kg per 24 hours = 50 mg/24 h
   - Calculate rate per hour: 50 mg/24 h = 2.1 mg/h
   - Calculate volume per hour: 2.1 mg/h ÷ 5 mg/mL = 0.42 mL/h of metoclopramide
   - Calculate how many hours of fluid therapy this bag will provide at rate of 100 mL/h: 1000 mL/100 mL per hour = 10 hours
   - Calculate volume of metoclopramide needed for 10-hour infusion: 10 hours × 0.42 mL/h = 4.2 mL
   - **4.2 mL metoclopramide should be added to 1000-mL bag.**

3. Calculate the rate according to patient weight: 5 kg × 0.2 mg/kg per hour = 1 mg/h
   - Calculate the volume per hour: 1 mg/h ÷ 10 mg/mL = 0.1 mL/h
   - Calculate how many hours the infusion will provide: 75 mL ÷ 15 mL/h = 5 hours
   - Calculate the volume of butorphanol needed for 5 hours: 0.1 mL/h × 5 hours = **0.5 mL of butorphanol to add to burette**

4. Calculate rate of KPO_4 according to patient weight: 12 kg × 0.02 mmol/kg per hour = 0.24 mmol/h KPO_4
   - Calculate volume of KPO_4: 0.24 mmol/h ÷ 3 mmol/mL = 0.08 mL/h KPO_4
   - Calculate how many hours of infusion: 150 mL ÷ 50 mL/h = 3 hours
   - Calculate total KPO_4 needed for 3-hour infusion: 3 hours × 0.08 mL/h = **0.24 mL KPO_4 to be added to burette**

It is necessary to calculate what K+ is contributed by this volume of KPO_4: 0.24 mL KPO_4 × 4.4 mEq K+/mL = 1.1 mEq K+

What is the equivalent of 1.1 mEq K+/150 mL in mEq/L?

- mEq K+/150 mL = x mEq K+/1000 mL = 7.3 mEq/L
- Calculate difference between 30 mEq K+/L and 7.3 mEq/L: 30 − 7.3 = 22.7 mEq/L
- This difference is made up by KCl supplement
- Calculate how many milliequivalents of K+ are needed to arrive at the concentration of 22.7 mEq/L in the 150-mL burette: 22.7/1000 = x/150 = (22.7 × 150 ÷ 1000) = x = 3.4 mEq K+ required from KCl
- Calculate volume of KCl required to give 3.4 mEq K+: 3.4 mEq ÷ 2 mEq/mL = **1.7 mL KCl to be added to burette**

5. Calculate rates according to patient weight:
   - Fentanyl: 43 kg × 3 µg/kg per hour = 129 µg/h
   - Volume of fentanyl = 129 µg/h ÷ 50 µg/mL = 2.6 mL/h
   - Ketamine: 43 kg × 0.2 mg/kg per hour = 8.6 mg/h
   - Volume of ketamine = 8.6 mg/h ÷ 100 mg/mL = 0.09 mL/h
   - Calculate number of hours of infusion in 1000-mL bag: 1000 mL ÷ 130 mL/h = 7.7 hours
   - Calculate volume of fentanyl and ketamine required for 7.7-hour infusion:
   - Volume of fentanyl = 2.6 mL/h × 7.7 hours = 20.0 mL fentanyl
   - Volume of ketamine = 0.09 mL/h × 7.7 hours = 0.69 mL ketamine
   - Because the volume of fentanyl to be added is fairly large, 20 mL of fluid should be removed before addition to maintain the same final volume

6a. Calculate the dose according to patient weight: 4 kg × 0.2 mg/kg per hour = 0.8 mg/h
   - Volume per hour = 0.8 mg/h ÷ 10 mg/mL = 0.08 mL/h
   - Calculate how many hours of infusion are in full burette: 150 mL ÷ 15 mL/h = 10 hours
   - Calculate volume of butorphanol needed for 10 hours: 10 hours × 0.08 mL/h = **0.8 mL butorphanol added to burette**

6b. Calculate the concentration of butorphanol in the burette: 0.8 mL of butorphanol × 10 mg/mL = 8 mg butorphanol in burette
   - 8 mg/150 mL = 0.05 mg/mL is concentration in burette
   - Calculate volume left in burette: 5 hours × 15 mL/h = 75 mL
   - Remaining volume in burette is 75 mL
   - Calculate number of hours of infusion in burette at new fluid rate: 75 mL ÷ 8 mL/h = 9.4 hours
   - Calculate butorphanol remaining in burette: 75 mL × 0.05 mg/mL = 3.75 mg butorphanol in burette
   - Prescribed dose of butorphanol was 0.8 mg/h (0.08 mL/h) butorphanol according to first calculations
   - Butorphanol required for remaining 9.4 hours: 9.4 hours × 0.8 mg/h = 7.52 mg
   - Currently have 3.75 mg butorphanol in burette but require 7.52
   - Calculate difference: 7.52 − 3.75 = 3.77 mg
   - 3.77 mg ÷ 10 mg/mL = **volume of butorphanol to be added = 0.37 mL**

6c. To halve the rate of the infusion of butorphanol that is currently in the burette, it is simplest to double the volume of fluid in the buretrol. **By adding 60 mL of fluid, the concentration of butorphanol, and hence the dose delivered, is decreased by half.**

7a. Calculate how many milligrams of dopamine are added to the bag: 5 mL × 40 mg/mL = 200 mg

- Calculate the concentration of the bag: 200 mg/250 mL = 0.8 mg/mL is the concentration of dopamine in the 250-mL bag
7b. 0.8 mg/mL × 1000 μg/1 mg = 800 μg/mL
7c. Calculate the rate according to the patient's weight: 6 μg/kg/min × 12 kg = 72 μg/min
    - Calculate the volume of dopamine: 72 μg/min ÷ 800 μg/mL = 0.09 mL/min
    - Calculate the volume per hour: 0.09 mL/min × 60 min/h = **5.4 mL/h is the rate of delivery of the dopamine solution**
8. Calculate the volume of the bolus with respect to the patient's weight: 15 kg × 15 mL/kg = **225 mL total volume of bolus and is set as the volume to be infused**
    - Calculate the fluid rate required to deliver 225 mL in 15 minutes
    - Fluid rate is programmed in milliliters per hour
    - 225 mL/15 min = x mL/60 min; solve for x
    - 225 × 60 ÷ 15 = **900 mL/h is the fluid rate required to deliver 225 mL over 15 minutes**
9a. Calculate the volume to be infused for the fluid bolus: 10 mL/kg × 12 kg = 120 mL
    - What fluid rate is needed to deliver 120 mL in 15 minutes:
    - x mL/60 min = 120 mL/15 min
    - Solve for x: 60 × 120 ÷ 15 = x; x = 480 mL/h
    - The pump should be set at a **rate of 480 mL/h** and a **volume to be infused of 120 mL** for the fluid bolus
9b. Calculate the patient's fluid deficit: 8/100 × 12 kg = **0.96 L or 960 mL** to be delivered over 24 hours.
    - The maintenance requirements for this dog are 12 × 50 = **600 mL/24 h**
    - Total volume to deliver over 24 hours = 960 mL + 600 mL = 1560 mL
    - Hourly rate = 1560 mL ÷ 24 hours = **65 mL/h is set as the rate on the pump for the fluid infusion over 24 hours.**

Review Questions

1. A dog receiving fluids at a rate of 55 mL/h is found to be hypokalemic on its most recent blood work. If the dog is prescribed fluids with 30 mEq KCl/L, how much KCl should be added to the 700 mL remaining in the fluid bag?
2. Calculate a constant rate infusion (CRI) of fentanyl (3 μg/kg per hour) for a 25-kg dog. How many milliliters of fentanyl does the dog receive per hour? The stock solution of fentanyl has a concentration of 50 μg/mL.
3. If no pumps, syringe drivers, or burettes are available, the fentanyl can be given by adding an appropriate volume to the bag. If the dog is receiving 75 mL/h of fluids and there are 600 mL left in bag, how much fentanyl should be added to the bag to provide the CRI above?
4. Your patient has been prescribed IV fluids with a 5% dextrose solution. How much dextrose should be added to a 100-mL burette to achieve this concentration? The stock solution of dextrose is a 50% solution.
5. The clinician has prescribed a metoclopramide infusion at 2 mg/kg per day for your 25-kg patient. The patient is receiving fluids at a rate of 50 mL/h. Assume that you are making up a 1-L bag of fluids for this patient and are required to put the medication directly into the bag. How much metoclopramide should you add to the bag?

Answers to the review questions can be found on page 223 in the Appendix. The review questions are also available for download on a companion website at www.wiley.com/ go/donohoenursing.

Further Reading

Bill, R. 2000. Percentages. In *Medical Mathematics and Dosage Calculations for Veterinary Professionals*, 97–110. Ames: Iowa State University Press.

Bill, R. 2000. Solving for the unknown value x. In *Medical Mathematics and Dosage Calculations for Veterinary Professionals*, 111–141. Ames: Iowa State University Press.

Mathews, K. 1996. Fluid therapy. In *Veterinary Emergency and Critical Care Manual*, 12-1–12-21. Guelph, Ontario, Canada: LifeLearn.

Mathews, K. 2006. Fluid therapy: non-hemorrhage. In *Veterinary Emergency and Critical Care Manual*, 347–372. Guelph, Ontario, Canada: LifeLearn.

Metheny, N. 1992. Intravenous therapy. In *Fluid and Electrolyte Balance: Nursing Considerations*, 149–168. Philadelphia: Lippincott.

Moore, M., and N. Palmer. 2001. Basic principles. In *Calculations for Veterinary Nurses*, 13–33. Oxford: Blackwell Science.

Moore, M., and N. Palmer. 2001. Changing the concentration of a solution. In *Calculations for Veterinary Nurses*, 33–55. Oxford: Blackwell Science.

Wanamaker, B., and K. Massey. 2004. Practical calculations in pharmacology. In *Applied Pharmacology for the Veterinary Technician*, 51–66. St. Louis: Saunders.

Patient Monitoring 6

Once a veterinary patient has been passed into the care of the technician, it is the technician's responsibility to become familiar with the patient. It is the technician's role to monitor every aspect of the patient's condition so he or she may be alerted to any changes that may interrupt the animal's convalescence.

Once technicians assume care of the patient, it behooves them to do their own assessment of the patient to determine their appreciation of the animal's current status. Some of the characteristics documented during a physical examination involve subjective appraisal. For example, what one person considers as pink mucous membranes may be considered by another as dark pink or injected. In addition, palpation of pulses may be difficult for one hospital staff member but not for another. The discrepancy between absent femoral pulses and easily palpable femoral pulses can lead to much confusion if it is not called into question until a time of crisis.

It is preferable for technicians to familiarize themselves with their patients as soon as care has been transferred. In so doing, much confusion may be avoided during times at which judgment is called into question.

Vital Signs

Vital signs are monitored every day in hospitalized patients. In the emergency or critical care setting, vitals are monitored several times a day and in some cases even hourly. By following trends in an animal's vital signs, the health care team is better able to predict when the animal's status is changing. This allows for more prompt reaction to any changes that arise.

Fluid Therapy for Veterinary Technicians and Nurses, First Edition. Charlotte Donohoe.
© 2012 Charlotte Donohoe. Published 2012 by John Wiley & Sons, Inc.

Vitals are measured using the caregiver's senses and abilities as well as using technical equipment. Despite the availability of highly specialized equipment, technicians must maintain their ability to monitor patients without relying heavily on electronic measurements. In the event that equipment malfunctions or delivers questionable results, technicians must be able to estimate the patient's condition relying solely on subjective measurements.

Temperature

Measurements of patients' body temperature are taken a minimum of twice daily in hospitalized animals. Intermittent monitoring can be performed much more frequently in patients that begin to show unexpected changes in temperature.

Measuring core body temperature is achieved through placement of a temperature sensor called a thermistor (Greer et al. 2007). The thermistor is placed in a body cavity that is centrally located within the patient's body. Placement in the esophagus is common in anesthetized patients. Thermistors may also be placed in the urinary bladder or in the pulmonary artery. Techniques required for placement of these catheters are invasive and time consuming. For these reasons, it is impractical to measure core body temperature in the private practice or critical care setting.

Critically ill patients may require continuous monitoring of body temperature. This technique is mainly reserved for patients that are anesthetized, mechanically ventilated, or at risk of overheating due to excessive work of breathing. Continuous monitoring is achieved by maintaining a flexible probe within the animal's rectum (Figs. 6.1 and 6.2). To stabilize the probe, tape may be fastened to the probe and anchored around the patient's tail. It is important not to secure the tape too tightly around the patient's tail in the event that circulation might be compromised.

Intermittent measurement of body temperature can be achieved by placement of a thermometer in the patient's rectum but may not be tolerated by some patients. In addition, this method may be inappropriate for some patients depending on the nature of

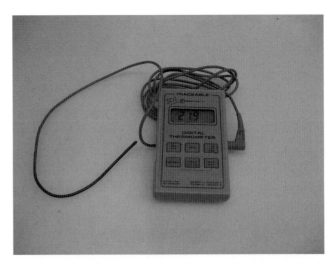

Figure 6.1.   Some patients require continuous monitoring of body temperature. Rectal temperature probes are well tolerated by most patients.

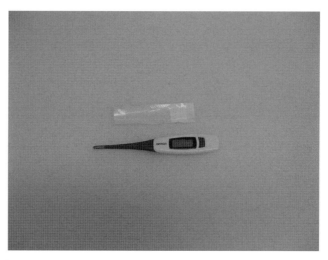

Figure 6.2. To reduce contamination between patients, disposable plastic sleeves should be used to cover thermometers before use. These are discarded after each use.

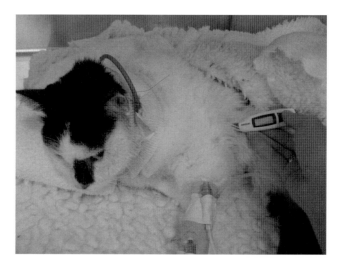

Figure 6.3. Thermometers placed well into the axilla provide a temperature comparable with rectal temperature in most patients. There is often a slightly lower temperature via axilla.

their illness. Patients that have undergone rectal surgery, have severe coagulopathies, or are extremely aggressive may not be ideal candidates for rectal thermometry. Rectal thermometry provides temperature values that closely resemble those of the body core (Greer et al. 2007). However, values may be erroneous if the thermometer fails to contact the mucosal surface and is instead inserted into a fecal ball.

Placement of the thermometer deep in a patient's axilla is well tolerated by most animals (Fig. 6.3). Measuring axillary temperature requires that the thermometer be held firmly under the patient's limb, ensuring it is at the most dorsal and proximal point possible.

Axillary temperatures must be evaluated with caution. Variations in temperature may be noted from one caregiver to the next depending on how the thermometer is positioned. Further, axillary temperatures do not consistently match rectal temperatures obtained at the same juncture in the same patient. Measurements taken from the axilla are of a slightly lower value than those obtained via rectum (Craig et al 2000).

Axillary temperature measurement can be used appropriately in patients whose temperatures have followed a stable trend and are unlikely to change with any degree of suddenness. Where accuracy is an absolute necessity, such as with patients at risk of infection or sepsis, ventilated patients, or patients with cardiac disease, it is a priority to have a reliable and repeatable temperature such as that obtained via rectal temperature (Greer et al. 2007).

Measurement of body temperature via infrared (IR) thermometer is another technique available to veterinary caregivers. The thermometer is covered in a thin plastic membrane inserted into the patient's ear. The device measures heat that radiates across the tympanic membrane. Due to the anatomic differences between humans and small animals, it is necessary to use an IR thermometer specifically designed for veterinary use. Due to the apparent fluctuation in reliability of these instruments, they have yet to gain commonplace status within the veterinary health care community.

Increases in body temperature

Normal body temperature for canine and feline patients most often lies between 37.5°C and 38.5°C. These animals can demonstrate mild fluctuations in body temperature prompted by the stress of merely being present in the veterinary hospital. Body temperature is considered elevated when it reaches 39.1°C.

Elevations in body temperature occur for many reasons. It is important for the technician to be familiar with possible causes of increased body temperature (i.e., infection, inflammation, excessive muscular activity) and to be able to differentiate between fever and hyperthermia.

Hyperthermia is the term that describes a patient whose body temperature is increased due to external causes. The increase in body temperature is not a defensive strike, as in the presence of infectious agents, but rather a result of the animal producing more body heat than it can effectively deal with. Patients in oxygen hoods or small cages, seizing patients, patients with severe muscle tremors, and respiratory distress patients whose work of breathing is excessive can all develop hyperthermia if not carefully monitored.

Generally speaking, hyperthermic patients are at a greater risk of developing body temperatures that are higher than pyrexic patients (Lagutchik 2002). Such high temperatures put the patient at risk for severe tissue injury and possibly death if the hyperthermia is not promptly reversed.

Febrile (pyrexic) patients have an elevated body temperature due to causes that exist within the patient's own body. Common causes of pyrexia include inflammation, infection, sepsis, neoplasia, and reaction to transfusion of blood product. Although any of these causes can lead to an extremely elevated body temperature, hyperthermic patients typically experience higher temperatures (Lagutchik 2002).

It is important to differentiate between hyperthermia and pyrexia because each condition is treated differently. Patients that are hyperthermic are responding to an environmental cause. As such, the technician is able to change the patient's environment and initiate cooling measures if the patient's body temperature is significantly elevated. Cooling should be initiated if the temperature exceeds 39.5°C (Mathews 2006b). Large patients benefit from large cage spaces or beds made up on the floor. Maximizing air circulation reduces the chances of patient overheating. If the patient's body temperature reaches dangerous levels, the patient will benefit from placement of a fan in relatively close proximity and may respond to the application of cool water. As body temperatures approach 41.0°C to 42.0°C, more aggressive measures are required. The patient's intravenous (IV) fluid line may be placed in a cool water bath. Further intervention may involve ice packs around the patient and infusion of room temperature saline into the bladder via a sterile urinary catheter. Flushing the bladder in this manner allows heat to transfer to the saline, which is then removed from the bladder via urinary catheter. The saline should remain in place for no longer than 5 minutes (Mathews 2006a). Active cooling should end once the patient's temperature has returned to approximately 39.0°C to 39.5°C (Walters 2002).

Patients that are pyrexic have an elevated body temperature that is a result of the body's attempts at defending itself. Temperatures reaching 41.0°C or higher require active cooling as just described. Temperatures below 41.0°C should be monitored closely but do not require active cooling. Providing this external cooling would make the patient's body work harder to maintain the higher temperature and thus use more of the patient's precious energy reserves. Pharmaceutical intervention with antipyretics or nonsteroidal anti-inflammatories is appropriate in pyrexic patients but inappropriate for hyperthermic patients (Walters 2002).

Decreases in body temperature

The term *hypothermia* refers to decreased body temperature. Normal body temperature for cats and dogs falls between 37.5°C and 38.5°C. A patient with a temperature below 37.5°C is hypothermic. Varying degrees of hypothermia are described as mild, moderate, and severe. The technician often encounters patients that fall in the category of mild hypothermia (34°C to 37°C) because postoperative patients and patients with heart failure generally fall within this range (Mathews 2006a).

Warming of a mildly to moderately hypothermic (30°C to 34°C) patient is achieved by providing a warm, dry environment for the animal. Warm blankets, oat bags (Fig. 6.4), circulating air or water blankets, water bottles, or microwaveable discs can be placed in close proximity to the patient to provide some additional heat (Figs. 6.4, 6.5, 6.6A, B, and 6.7). It is imperative that none of the external heat sources are in contact with the patient's skin. Thermal burns are a devastating consequence of heating instruments being placed against a patient's skin.

When monitoring a hypothermic patient, the technician must be constantly aware of other vital parameters. Mentation, heart rate, blood pressure, and mucous membrane color are all affected by decreased body temperature.

Severely hypothermic (28°C to 30°C) patients require more invasive monitoring and rewarming techniques (Mathews 2006a). Lavage of urinary bladder or of pleural space or peritoneal cavity with warm sterile saline or dialysis fluid, respectively, is an extreme measure reserved for patients that are severely hypothermic and/or cardiovascularly unstable (Mathews 2006a; Wingfield 2002).

Heart Rate

Heart rate (HR) can be measured via several different routes. The simplest of these is palpation of pulses. This is an extremely noninvasive procedure that is well tolerated by most patients. One of the benefits of palpating pulses is that it can be performed on

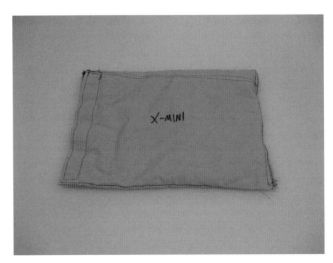

Figure 6.4. Microwaveable oat bags can be used to rewarm patients. They should never be placed directly against the animal's skin.

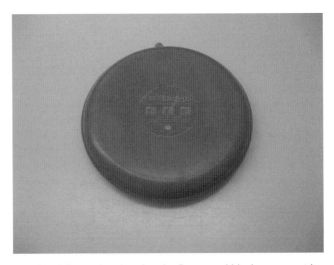

Figure 6.5. Microwaveable disks can be placed under fleeces and blankets to provide warm housing.

a recumbent patient with little disturbance to the animal. A true resting HR can sometimes be noted if the animal remains stress free and allows easy access to its femoral or dorsal pedal pulses. Weak or absent pulses immediately alert the technician to the fact that the animal needs prompt attention and intervention. This type of instant evaluation yields more information than measurement of HR by any other means. Poor pulse quality can indicate hypovolemia, hypotension, hypothermia, and several other types of dysfunction. In this regard, monitoring HR using pulses provides additional information that is not obtained by simple auscultation or electrocardiogram (ECG) monitoring.

HR can also be measured via thoracic auscultation (Fig. 6.8). Auscultation depends on the use of a stethoscope but is a reliable means of obtaining an HR. This procedure may be subject to technical difficulty if the patient is experiencing an abnormal accumulation of fluid in the pleural or pericardial space.

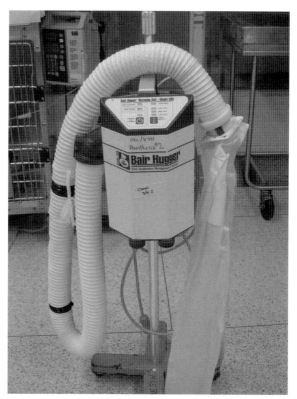

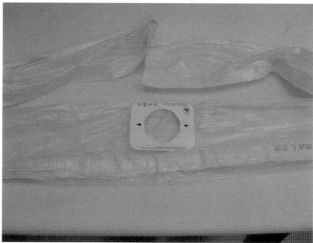

Figure 6.6. Bair huggers circulate warm air around the patient and rewarm animals with less risk of iatrogenic thermal injury.

Measurement of HR is also achievable via ECG. A patient may be connected to an intermittent or continuous ECG for monitoring of HR and rhythm. For the sake of patient comfort, it is preferable to shave small areas of fur and place ECG pads on the patient's skin (Fig. 6.9). The adhesive pads have small buttons to which ECG leads are clipped to facilitate measurement of rate and rhythm. It is important that the gel pad

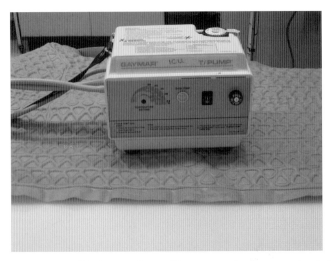

Figure 6.7. Circulating hot water blankets can be used for patients that cannot maintain body temperature.

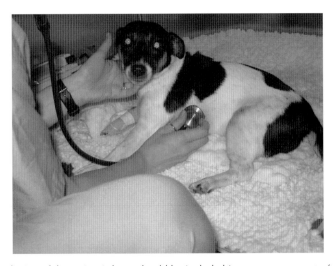

Figure 6.8. Auscultation of the patient's heart should be included in every assessment of a new patient.

(surrounded by the adhesive material) is in complete contact with the patient's skin. Interruptions in this contact can lead to artifact or absence of ECG tracing.

Artifact can also be the result of patient movement or loose connections between the patient and the lead or between the lead and the machine. If difficulty is encountered during the technician's attempts to obtain an ECG tracing, these problem areas should be investigated promptly because they are often easily corrected.

Many different situations can cause a change in patient HR. If the technician observes a sudden change in HR that is not explained by exercise or a change in position, the change warrants further investigation.

A patient's HR changes in response to several conditions. Any change in HR warrants evaluation of other vital signs to determine whether they have been affected as well.

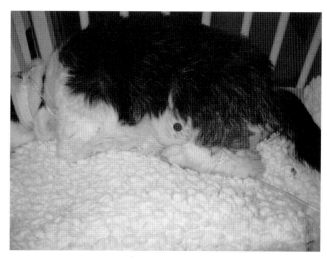

Figure 6.9. Animals expected to be on continuous ECG monitors benefit from placement of adhesive pads rather than clips.

Tachycardia

As the technician monitors a patient, changes in HR may occur in subtle or dramatic forms. Increases in HR and progression to tachycardia (accelerated heart rate) can be the result of physiologic changes that a patient is undergoing throughout an illness.

The technician can develop a repertoire that includes causes of tachycardia to be investigated once an elevation in HR is noted. Other vital parameters should be measured as part of the investigation.

One of the simplest causes to investigate is pain. Assuming the patient is cardiovascularly stable and that hypovolemia and hypoxia have been dismissed as potential causes for tachycardia, the technician may administer a cautious dose of analgesics. The animal's reaction to the analgesics will allow the technician to quickly determine whether or not pain is the cause of the elevated HR. If the patient's HR decreases and the patient seems to respond positively to the dose of analgesics, the likely cause of the change in HR was pain.

Anxiety may also be a cause of elevated HR. A large and important part of the technician's role is to provide a comfortable, clean, stress-free environment for hospital patients. If all comforts have been provided and the patient's anxiety level is still very high, it may be necessary to offer some mild sedation to ensure that the patient does not do itself any detriment.

Decreased tissue oxygenation is also a cause of HR elevation. Distribution of oxygenated blood is carried out in part by arterial blood flow. Presuming that red blood cells are being appropriately bound with oxygen as they travel through the lungs, the forward motion provided by the heart should distribute adequate levels of oxygen to the remainder of the body. In times of low tissue oxygenation, HR can increase to augment cardiac output (CO) (recall that $CO = HR \times$ stroke volume). This is an extremely simplified version of what transpires, but it is meant to illustrate that hypoxia can be a cause of tachycardia.

Hypovolemia is another common cause of tachycardia. Receptors throughout the vasculature sense that vascular volume is below what is optimal for the particular animal. Through a series of complex events, the body responds by attempting to increase cardiac output. As with the example mentioned earlier, one of the ways in which the body can increase CO is to increase HR.

A hypovolemic patient may present with tachycardia or may develop tachycardia if its volume status is not appropriately maintained throughout its illness. Fluid therapy, possibly aggressive fluid therapy, may be necessary to counter the effects of hypovolemia. Clinician's orders may include a fluid bolus followed closely by reevaluation of the patient's vital signs. If the fluid bolus provides some degree of relief from the hypovolemia, it should be indicated by an associated decrease in HR. If many physiologic factors are contributing to the patient's tachycardia, there may not be as notable a response to the fluid bolus. Slight improvements in HR and volume status may be perpetuated with additional fluid boluses, provided each is followed by a thorough assessment of the patient's vitals and its response to the fluid bolus.

Hypokalemia, another potential cause for increases in HR, is also treated by means of fluid therapy. Should arrhythmias arise as a result of hypokalemia, they will be reflected by an increase in HR, possibly irregular pulses, and abnormal heart sounds may be noted on auscultation. Potassium supplementation is necessary in severely affected patients to avoid the development of cardiac arrhythmias.

Hypercarbia, toxin ingestion, hyperthermia, cardiac arrhythmias, and heart failure are also causes of elevations in HR. Causes of tachycardia can be relatively benign, such as with stress; or extremely dangerous, such as with an arrhythmia. It is imperative that the technician monitor a patient's heart rate with all of these possibilities in mind. Any increase in HR should be fully investigated.

Bradycardia

Bradycardia refers to a heart rate that is slower than what is normally expected for a given patient. In the emergency and critical care setting, this condition is often appreciated at time of presentation of a patient. This is in contrast to tachycardia, which may develop for a variety of reasons at any point during the patient's illness. Although a hospitalized patient may develop bradycardia during its illness, I would argue that the opposite is more common.

Causes of bradycardia include but are not limited to hyperkalemia, hypocalcemia, toxin ingestion, and increased intracranial pressure. Patients suffering from any one of these conditions will benefit, if not absolutely require, hospitalization and support that includes fluid therapy. However, fluid therapy does not play the same role in bradycardic patients as it does with tachycardic patients. With respect to hypovolemia, tachycardic patients have a significant need for fluid to augment their volume status. The result is that once the volume has been replenished, the heart does not need to work as fast to circulate the blood volume. It is much less common to be in a situation where the effects of fluid therapy reverse bradycardia. Treatment of bradycardia is usually achieved with pharmaceutical intervention, often including the use of electrolyte therapy.

Respiratory Rate

Respiratory rate (RR) is measured in the conscious patient by counting the number of chest excursions that the patient has within a certain time frame. Regardless of the time period used to count breaths, the RR is documented in breaths per minute.

During a physical examination, respiratory rate may be counted via thoracic auscultation. Auscultation is performed to evaluate the patient's heart and lung sounds, but it may be used to obtain an RR as well. This is not the easiest method for counting RR, however.

Counting RRs in anxious or active patients may be difficult to accomplish. It is best to monitor RR a slight distance away from the patient where possible. When RR is evaluated at time of presentation, for example as a part of a triage examination, the technician may choose to count the RR while the patient is being held by the owner. If this is accomplished before the technician approaches the patient, there is a better chance that the animal's RR will not yet be elevated as a result of anxiety. In large dogs that are not able to be held by the owner, it is still advisable for the technician to count RR from a distance where possible. In many cases, the canine patient is curious enough that sniffing of furniture and floor space will hinder the acquisition of a true RR.

In the hospital setting, approaching the kennel without opening the door and without alerting the patient is a means by which the technician can get a true representation of the patient's respiratory pattern at rest.

In addition to monitoring RR, the technician must be well versed in monitoring respiratory noises and patterns. Becoming familiar with thoracic auscultation and which sounds are normal for healthy patients is a requirement of the emergency and critical care technician.

Patients that develop moist lung sounds, crackles, or wheezes may do so as a result of excessive administration of fluid therapy.

Tachypnea

Tachypnea is the term used to describe an abnormally elevated respiratory rate. *Dyspnea* is the term used to describe a patient that is having difficulty breathing. Dsypnea is often accompanied by tachypnea, but tachypnea can be present alone. Causes of tachypnea are numerous; the technician should be familiar with common causes in the event that multiple forms of intervention are necessary.

Tachypneic or distressed patients should immediately be placed in an oxygen-rich environment or have oxygen administered via flow by or via nasal cannula. Providing oxygen to the tachypneic patient affords the patient care team the time to investigate possible causes of the tachypnea.

Common causes of tachypnea include but are not limited to primary lung disease, pleural space disease, anemia, pain, anxiety, and neurologic disease. Anxious or painful patients are unlikely to show changes in clinical signs despite the addition of oxygen to their environment, which may help caregivers determine the true cause of the patient's tachypnea. Conversely, a patient that is tachypneic due to hypoxia should demonstrate a slight decrease in RR once supplemental oxygen is provided.

Additional monitoring with pulse oximetry is helpful in tachypneic patients. Portable pulse oximeters are available in most veterinary hospitals and used with frequency and confidence (Fig. 6.10). They do not require a great degree of technical skill and are well tolerated by most patients. Pulse oximeters measure patient HR and the percentage of hemoglobin that is saturated with oxygen in arterial blood. Normal ranges for healthy patients breathing room air are expected to fall between 95% and 100%. Oxygen supplementation is recommended if the saturation of oxygen (SpO_2) drops to 92% or less (Hammond and Walters 1999).

Patients receiving long-term fluid therapy should be monitored closely for signs of increasing respiratory rates. Pulmonary edema and pleural effusion are possible

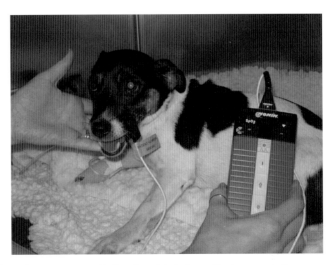

Figure 6.10. Pulse oximeters are practical and useful during patient assessment.

complications associated with fluid volume overload (Rudloff and Kirby 2001). Both of these conditions lead to elevated respiratory rates and difficulty breathing. Prompt intervention is needed to reverse the effects of fluid overload. For these reasons, the technician must be diligent with respect to monitoring respiratory rates of fluid therapy patients.

Bradypnea

Bradypnea is the term describing a respiratory rate that is abnormally low. This condition is not as frequently encountered as tachypnea. Complications related to fluid therapy rarely, if ever, result in bradypnea.

Common causes of decreased RR include narcotic administration, toxin ingestion, and increased intracranial pressure. In severe cases, where the patient's RR is low enough to compromise tissue oxygenation, mechanical ventilation may be required.

Bradypneic patients may require fluid therapy to support them through the particular crisis that has them hospitalized. Fluids may be used for the purpose of diuresis, drug administration, or simply to provide the animal's maintenance fluid requirement during a period of diminished health.

Body Weight

Patients receiving fluid therapy must undergo a minimum of once-daily measurement of body weight. Emergency and critical care patients should optimally be weighed at least twice daily and, in some circumstances, more frequently than that.

Weight measurements are achieved in many different ways depending on the type of equipment available to the technician. Many veterinary practices benefit from large walk-on scales that are excellent for use with most canine patients (Fig. 6.11).

Feline patients and some small or toy canine breeds may be difficult to assess using the large floor scales. For these patients it may be less of a challenge to weigh the animal

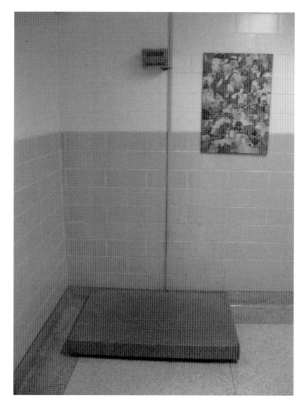

Figure 6.11. A floor scale is a convenient way to weigh large ambulatory patients.

in a carrier or while they are being carried by a caregiver. If the caregiver stands on the scale with the patient, the caregiver's weight is subtracted from the total to provide the current weight of the patient.

Small tabletop scales are most accurate for small patients and tend to be slightly less daunting for these animals because many of the scales have raised sides that provide a sense of security (Fig. 6.12).

An important consideration while trending body weight is that the patient be weighed on the same scale each time a weight is obtained. This eliminates the possibility of inadvertent misinterpretation of weight changes that can arise using two scales that are calibrated differently (Fig. 6.13).

Monitoring changes in body weight provides a means of determining whether the patient is retaining any of the fluid being delivered throughout its therapy. It is widely accepted that 1 kg of body weight represents 1 L of fluid (DiBartola 2006). It follows that a loss or gain of 0.5 kg (500 g) over a short period of time represents a loss or gain of 500 mL.

Fluid gains and losses are also monitored through urinary output; however, body weight is a simple and fast method of estimating a patient's response to fluid therapy. It is important to consider the goal of the fluid therapy so that changes in body weight can be appropriately evaluated. For example, a patient receiving fluids due to dehydration and hypovolemia should gain weight as the fluid deficit is replaced. This weight gain is expected. In contrast, a patient suffering from septic peritonitis may experience a weight gain that exceeds what is expected of this patient. In sepsis, several physiologic

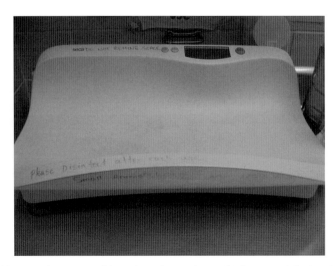

Figure 6.12. Tabletop scales are portable and can be used in multiple areas of the hospital to weigh small patients.

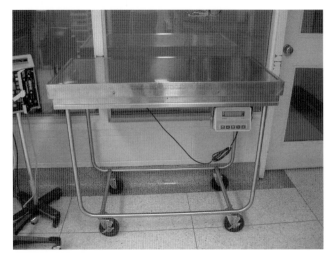

Figure 6.13. A mobile scale can be used for small and medium-size patients and can double as a treatment table.

changes take place that have widespread consequences for the patient. For example, the capillaries can sustain damage and become overly permeable. Proteins leak through these capillaries, escape the vasculature, and leak into the tissues. This shift causes the colloid osmotic pressure to decrease in the vessels and increase in the tissue. The increased number of proteins in the tissue attracts body water and draws it into the tissue space. As fluid leaves the vasculature and flows toward the tissues, the patient may become hypovolemic despite fluid therapy. The fluid that is leaked into the tissue space accumulates and causes a temporary weight gain in the patient (DiBartola 2006). This is sometimes referred to as "third spacing."

As the condition of the septic patient improves, the capillaries become less permeable and eventually return to normal. Subsequently, protein levels within the vasculature also return to normal. Fluid that had leaked into the tissues eventually shifts back into the vasculature, drawn there by the reinstated colloid osmotic pressure. This massive fluid shift back into the vascular space leads to a dramatic increase in urine output. Although the patient is still receiving fluid therapy, the urinary losses typically exceed the volume that is gained through IV therapy. The overall result is that the patient undergoes weight loss.

Recall that serial measurement of body weight is reflective of fluid lost or gained through therapy if the change in body weight occurs over a short period of time (such as 12 hours).

Central Venous Pressure

Central venous pressure is a parameter measured via a catheter placed into a central vein. The tip of the catheter must lie within the proximal or the caudal vena cava to be able to measure CVP. Measurement is achieved through one of several methods (Tables 6.1 and 6.2). Hospitals that benefit from the availability of advanced monitoring systems have the capacity to measure CVP using an electronic transducer and computer that calculates CVP and displays it on a digital monitor (Fig. 6.14). Simpler methods involve the use of a manometer and a fluid line, a technique that is within the means of most veterinary practices (Fig. 6.15, and 6.16A, B). Hospitals that do not have access to a manometer may also fashion a homemade version using a fluid line and a ruler.

CVP measurement allows the health care team to monitor the effects of fluid therapy with a great degree of insight. Placement of the catheter within the proximal vena cava provides an estimation of the pressure within the right atrium. For the purpose of this description we can consider this point to be the beginning point of the cardiac cycle. It fits that in knowing the pressure that exists at this point we have a sense of the volume of blood arriving at the heart. The blood that arrives at the heart to begin another cycle through the cardiovascular system is referred to as *preload*.

CVP measurements are not solely interpreted with respect to volume and preload, but they are also reflective of cardiac function. For example, an elevation in CVP may be explained by an increase in circulating volume, but it may also be a reflection of the heart's inability to provide forward momentum. A decrease in the heart's ability to pump blood in a forward direction would also result in elevation in pressure within the right atrium and proximal vena cava.

Table 6.1   Technique for Central Venous Pressure Measurement Using Manometer

- Fluid line primed and connected to central venous catheter
- Other end of fluid line connected to three-way stopcock
- Stopcock connected to manometer
- Manometer connected to fluid line that is connected to fluid bag
- 0 measurement on manometer is at level of right atrium
- Line is primed while stopcock is *off* to patient
- Manometer is filled
- Stopcock opened to patient
- Fluid level in manometer drops while pressure equalizes with central venous pressure
- Level of fluid in manometer is central venous pressure reading

Table 6.2 Measurement of Central Venous Pressure Using Electronic Transducer

- Lines are primed before connection
- Rigid fluid line connected to central venous catheter
- Opposite end of rigid line connected to transducer
- Fluid line from transducer to fluid bag
- Transducer is turned off to patient and machine is calibrated to zero
- Stopcock turned off to fluid bag
- Transducer measures pressure change
- Computer cable from transducer to monitoring hardware transfers information that is then displayed in wave and numeric form on screen

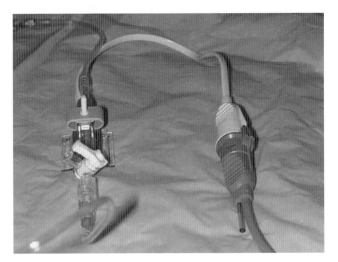

Figure 6.14. A transducer converts information obtained from blood pressure measurement and relays it to a computer monitor for display of patient parameters.

CVP measurements must be taken throughout the course of fluid therapy to observe the patient's response to fluids at different intervals. The benefits of CVP monitoring are derived from observing trends for each patient rather than using a single measurement. This is in part due to the fact that the chambers of the heart are compliant to a certain degree and can accommodate changes in circulating volume without eliciting a change in CVP that is measurable at a given point in time (Spiess and Gomez 1998). By repeating measurements, the technician is able to record a range of values for each patient and be well aware when a specific change is outside the acceptable range for that animal.

CVP is measured in two different units: cm H_2O or mm Hg. To convert mm Hg to cm H_2O, the value obtained in mm Hg is multiplied by a factor of 1.36 to obtain cm H_2O. A range of 0 to 10 cm H_2O is accepted as normal for canine and feline patients (deLaforcade and Rozanski 2001). Although a value that falls within this range is considered normal, it is most important to obtain a measurement for the individual patient that is defined as a starting point. In so doing, the technician is able to reevaluate the patient's CVP and know in which direction it has progressed as the patient has received fluids.

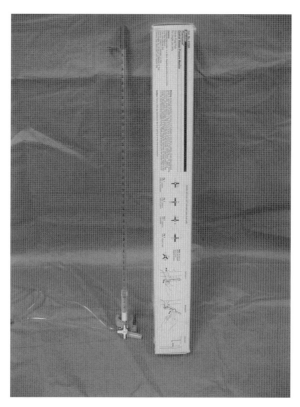

Figure 6.15. CVP can be measured using a manometer. This method does not require special or computerized equipment.

Decreased CVP

It is common that patients who present with a history of several days of anorexia, vomiting, and/or diarrhea show signs of hypovolemia or hypovolemic shock during the initial physical examination. These patients are perceived to have a decreased circulating volume within their vasculature that can be confirmed through the use of CVP measurement. IV access and fluid therapy should be initiated immediately to counter the effects of severe hypovolemia. At a point that it is appropriate to do so (available technical personnel, decrease in clinical signs of hypovolemic shock, palpable or visible central venous access) a central line can be placed for measurement of CVP.

The CVP of a volume-depleted patient most often falls below the normal range and is less than 0 cm H_2O (deLaforcade and Rozanski 2001). While the patient is volume resuscitated, the technician can monitor CVP and guide fluid therapy according to the patient's response. One or several fluid boluses may be required before the CVP rises above 0 cmH_2O. Severely volume-depleted patients may not display a change in CVP until multiple boluses are administered. Provided that the patient is not experiencing any degree of cardiac disease, a goal of an increase of 2 to 4 cm H_2O is appropriate (Hansen 2006). If continued measurement reflects an immediate return to the baseline value, the circulating volume has still not been augmented to a suitable level. Resuscitative efforts (fluid boluses) should continue until the increase in CVP takes slightly longer to return to its baseline value. A 15-minute guideline for return to initial CVP is reflective of a near normal circulating volume and successful volume resuscitation (Mathews 2006c).

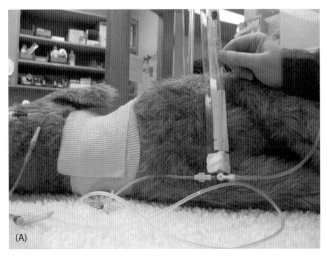

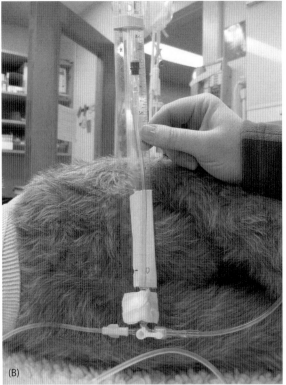

Figure 6.16. (A) For CVP measurement, a manometer can be devised using a fluid line and a ruler. (B) The zero point on the ruler is positioned at the level of the right atrium.

Increased CVP

Elevations in CVP reflect in increase in the volume of blood returning to the right atrium or an increase in the pressure within this chamber. Animals suffering from heart disease have a diminished capacity to propel blood forward through the heart.

Another situation in which pressure rises in the proximal vena cava occurs when a patient is the recipient of overzealous fluid administration.

Patients with heart disease and patients receiving fluid therapy for several days are at greater risk for volume overload (deLaforcade and Rozanski 2001). CVP measurements should be obtained several times daily in these patients so the technician is promptly alerted to trends showing increasing values. Significantly elevated CVPs (>10 cm H_2O) are reflective of volume overload that can put the patient at risk of pulmonary edema (Hansen 2006).

Nursing considerations

Proper technique is the cornerstone of accurate CVP measurement. One of the most important considerations is the placement of the 0 point of the measurement system. Regardless of whether a ruler, manometer, or transducer is in use, the zero point must lie as close to the right atrium as possible. To position this point correctly, the technician can use the following landmarks:

- If the patient is lying in lateral recumbency, the right atrium is estimated to be at the level of the manubrium
- If the patient is lying in sternal recumbency, the right atrium is estimated to be at the level of the scapulohumeral joint

When recording CVP measurements the technician should also record which position the patient was in at the time of measurement, including whether the lateral recumbency was right or left.

As with any measurement made using an intravascularly placed catheter, complications may arise if the catheter becomes kinked or clotted. The technician can improve efficiency by flushing the catheter before measurement to ensure the CVP reading is not affected by catheter obstruction. In addition, if other fluids are being delivered into the same catheter, it is imperative that all other ports and lines be clamped at the most proximal point. The only port that should remain open is the one being used for the CVP measurement, and it should be the most proximal port possible. The line distal to this port is also clamped and its infusion is temporarily suspended. It is prudent to verify that all connections and wires are securely connected if an electronic transducer is in use.

Blood Pressure

Measuring blood pressure is achieved via several different methods. Different equipment is required depending on which method is selected; choice may be made based on practice type, cost, and availability of technically skilled hospital personnel. Each blood pressure measurement system has advantages and drawbacks, and there is some variability with respect to accuracy.

Indirect blood pressure measurement

Obtaining an indirect BP involves the use of either a Doppler or an oscillometric blood pressure measurement system (Figs. 6.17 and 6.18). The Doppler method uses a small probe that contains a crystal that senses the movement of blood flow when placed over a peripheral artery. The probe is accompanied by a speaker through which the sound of the flow is rendered audible to the operator. Flow is temporarily obstructed by inflation of a cuff placed proximal to the probe. A sphygmomanometer is used to inflate the cuff and subsequently slowly deflate the cuff. The pressure reading is made when the whooshing sound of blood flow becomes audible once again. The pressure obtained by a Doppler is the *systolic* blood pressure of the patient.

The Doppler probe is positioned after a small patch of fur is clipped over an accessible artery and contact between the skin and the probe is facilitated by application of gel. It is important that the technician is aware of the pressure being applied to the probe; only gentle pressure is necessary to maintain proper positioning over the artery. If the technician applies a significant amount of pressure, it may be impossible to appreciate any sound at all. Further difficulty may arise if the patient is hypothermic. Cold temperatures cause a decrease in peripheral circulation, and as such, arterial flow is diminished and occasionally difficult to hear with a Doppler. When the patient's blood pressure is extremely low, it may be impossible to obtain a reading with the Doppler.

Oscillometric pressure measurements are made using an electronic machine that provides numeric results in digital format. A cuff is also used with this style of blood pressure measurement and is attached to the mechanical inflator rather than a manual one. Cuff size influences the results obtained with each reading. The technician should select cuff size with care and try to use cuffs whose *widths* are approximately 40%–60% of the limb circumference. Selection of a cuff that is too small will cause artificial elevation of blood pressure. Too generous a cuff size will provide a pressure that is falsely low (Waddell 2004).

Oscillometric measurement is a very complex procedure. The following is a simplified description of the processes involved. The oscillometric machine occludes the patient's artery by inflating the cuff with air. The machine senses the return of blood flow as it releases the air pressure within the cuff. As the artery oscillates with the flow of blood, the systolic blood pressure is measured. The diastolic pressure is measured at the point at which the oscillations quickly become insensible. Mean arterial pressure (MAP) is the blood pressure at which the oscillations reach their widest amplitude (Waddell 2004).

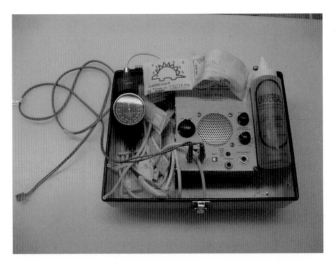

Figure 6.17.   Doppler blood pressure measurement is often more easily achieved in smaller patients than oscillometric blood pressure.

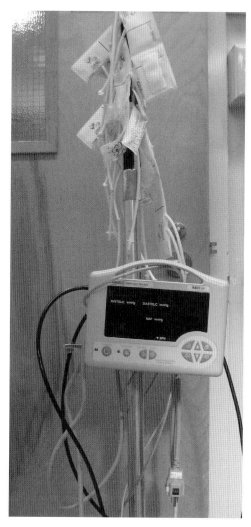

Figure 6.18. Oscillometric blood pressure measurement is a type of indirect blood pressure measurement. Cuff size is selected according to patient size.

Patient position is an important consideration when measuring BP via the oscillometric method. The cuff should be positioned in close proximity to the level of the heart. It is preferable to have the patient in sternal or lateral recumbency to achieve this goal. Patient movement will interfere with the machine's ability to distinguish the true motion of the artery and will result in artificial values.

Most oscillometric blood pressure equipment also provides a value for the patient's HR. The machine has the ability to count the number of oscillations of the artery that occur in a minute and will provide a reasonable estimate of heart rate in ideal conditions.

Direct arterial measurement

Direct arterial blood pressure (DABP) measurement is regarded as the most accurate way of monitoring blood pressure (Fig. 6.19A, B). It is more technically challenging

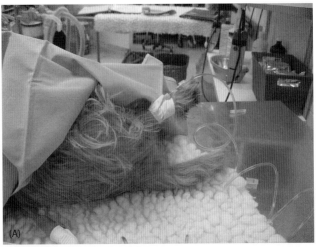

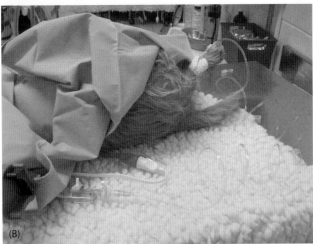

Figure 6.19. (A) Direct arterial pressure measurement is obtained via an arterial catheter in the hind limb. A rigid fluid line is connected to the catheter, through the PRN Adapter, and then to a transducer and pressurized fluid bag. (B) The transducer (lower left by the sterile lap sheet) converts information regarding the pressure changes it senses and conveys the information to the computer.

than indirect methods but yields more information and is thus suitable for more intensive patients.

Placement of an arterial catheter is the foundation for DABP monitoring. This procedure is similar to that for placement of a venous catheter. Arterial catheter placement is slightly more of a challenge due to the reactive potential of the arterial wall once it is invaded by the catheter. The walls of the arteries are more muscular than those of other vessels and can tightly constrict around the catheter, making it difficult to advance off the stylet. Another challenge encountered with arterial catheterization is the difficulty with which the vessels themselves are visualized. Whereas a vein is often easily visualized, raised, and palpated, an artery is not occluded and does not visibly rise when filled with blood. The arteries are palpable and once the pulse has been identified, a location for catheter placement may be selected.

Arterial catheters may be secured in the same fashion as venous catheters. Heparinized saline flushes are required with greater frequency in arterial catheters than with venous; every 2 hours is adequate to maintain arterial line patency.

The equipment required for measurement of DABP may be cost prohibitive to some practices. Many of the machines available for this purpose also measure CVP, ECG, end tidal carbon dioxide, and in some cases even pulmonary capillary wedge pressure (Fig. 6.20). To measure DABP, a rigid fluid line with a sterile hypodermic needle at its end is inserted into the injection port/Luer adapter that is secured to the arterial catheter. The line is connected to a pressure transducer, which is then connected to another fluid line and pressurized fluid bag via a three-way stopcock. The transducer is also connected to the electronic monitor via computer cable. As with the configuration of lines for CVP measurement, the transducer should be maintained at the level of the patient's heart. The stopcock is turned off to the patient while the monitor is calibrated to zero. Once this is achieved, the stopcock is opened to the patient and the transducer interprets and conveys the arterial pressure to the monitor where it is displayed.

Critically ill patients benefit from continuous monitoring of arterial blood pressure because their condition can change with such rapidity. If the monitoring is continuous, it is still prudent to flush the arterial catheter from time to time to ensure patency. Table 6.3 lists the advantages and disadvantages associated with the different methods of blood pressure measurement.

Hypotension

Hypotension is appreciated in many emergency and critical care patients. It is defined as a MAP below 60 mm Hg. Various culprits may be responsible for the patient's low blood pressure. Hypovolemia, bradycardia, sepsis, and hemorrhage are some common causes of hypotension. Another common cause of hypotension is anesthesia.

As a patient's blood pressure drops, perfusion to tissues and organs is compromised. At MAPs below 60 mm Hg, perfusion to the kidneys and brain is inadequate.

Hypotension can be treated by providing intravascular volume through fluid administration. It is the clinician's responsibility to determine what volume of fluid can safely be administered in any given situation and how quickly it should be delivered. Choices for volume expansion are not limited to crystalloids but can include synthetic colloids, natural colloids, and/or additional blood products. Fluid therapy plays a vital role in treating many causes of hypotension.

Hypotension in the face of fluid intervention may indicate the need for pharmaceutical therapy such as vasopressors or positive inotropes (Mathews 2006e).

Hypertension

Hypertension is defined as an elevated blood pressure and used to describe a patient whose systolic blood pressure is greater than 145 mm Hg (deLaforcade and Rozanski 2001). Disease processes leading to hypertension include renal disease, hyperthyroidism, pheochromocytoma, and neoplasia.

Fluid therapy is often used as part of the overall intervention for hypertensive patients, but it is not a specific treatment. Most causes of hypertension require pharmaceutical intervention and/or removal of the primary cause.

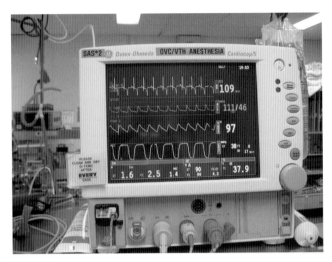

Figure 6.20. The waveform of the direct arterial pressure is second down from the top. The blood pressure measurement is read at the right side. Note that each wave spike in the arterial pressure corresponds with a complex on the ECG (an increase in pressure follows each contraction).

Table 6.3 Advantages and Disadvantages Associated with Different Methods of Blood Pressure Medication

Method of Blood Pressure Measurement	Advantages	Disadvantages
Doppler	<ul><li>Relatively inexpensive</li><li>Portable</li><li>Accurate</li><li>Sensitive enough to read low pressures</li><li>Ability to determine pressure in presence of arrhythmia</li></ul>	<ul><li>Only provides systolic pressure</li><li>Debates exist with respect to adding 10 mm Hg to pressures in cats</li><li>Difficult to hear in noisy or busy hospital setting</li></ul>
Oscillometric	<ul><li>Minimal technical ability needed</li><li>Provides systolic, diastolic, mean arterial pressure, and heart rate</li><li>Repeat pressure measurement available at preselected intervals</li><li>Alarm settings for pressures outside normal range</li></ul>	<ul><li>Cost</li><li>Poor reliability with patient movement, arrhythmia, hypothermia, vasoconstriction</li></ul>
Direct arterial	<ul><li>Considered most accurate method</li><li>Means of continuous blood pressure monitoring</li><li>Allows for waveform analysis</li></ul>	<ul><li>Technical expertise required for placement of arterial catheter</li><li>Cost of monitoring equipment, transducer</li><li>Catheter maintenance</li><li>Invasive procedure for patient (catheter placement)</li></ul>

Urine Output

Monitoring urine output in hospitalized patients can provide additional information that is useful in the management of fluid therapy. Whether the patient is nonambulatory and requires a urinary catheter or can manage to urinate outdoors or in a litter box, the technician may collect urine to evaluate volume and urine specific gravity (USG). Evaluation of these parameters imparts knowledge about the patient's volume status in that the volume of urine output can be partly predicted once the patient's deficit has been replaced.

Animals receiving fluid therapy are expected to produce a minimum of 1 to 2 mL/kg per hour (DiBartola 2006) of urine if renal function is adequate. The hourly volume of urine produced by a patient is calculated by the technician over a set period of time. During this time period all of the patient's urine should be collected. This calculation is more readily achieved if a 24-hour time period is broken into 4- or 6-hour intervals. If a 20-kg dog urinates 200 mL every 4 hours, that dog is passing 50 mL/h, which satisfies the minimum requirement of 20 to 40 mL/h for this patient.

Urine collection can be carried out via several different methods. Consideration should be given to the nature of the illness of the patient and the patient's ability to ambulate when decided on the means for urine collection. Free catch or free flow urine may be obtained from most canine patients if they are able to walk outside. The fact that this sample may be contaminated by the environment is a drawback associated with this method of collection. In addition, it may be difficult to capture the entire volume of urine being passed as the dog may hesitate or may knock the collection container while posturing to urinate.

Where animals choose to urinate on bedding, the bedding may be weighed before placement in the kennel and then again once it has been urinated on. The difference in weight can be used to estimate the volume of urine excreted. A total of 100 g of urine is approximately equal to 100 mL. Urine measurements in feline patients can be facilitated through the use of a nonabsorbent material in the litter box.

Another option for small but ambulatory patients is the use of a metabolic cage. These cages have a slanted bottom with a drain in the center. A collection system is placed under the drain to collect any urine that is passed in the kennel. The patient rests on a flat elevated grate and passes urine through the grate if inclined to urinate in the kennel. Collection and interpretation of urine production can be compromised if the patient manages to spill the water bowl because that liquid will also collect in the system underneath the kennel.

Patients that are nonambulatory, that are at risk of urine scald, or that require intensive monitoring of urine output (as with renal failure patients) are candidates for indwelling transurethral urinary catheters. Placement of urinary catheters in both male and female cats and dogs is a procedure that requires a moderate amount of technical expertise. However, with appropriate knowledge, guidance, and practice, the veterinary technician is able to perform this procedure readily in most patients.

One of the reasons that urine output is measured is so it can be compared with the volume of fluid that has been delivered to the patient during the course of its fluid therapy. This is an additional means by which fluid therapy can be monitored. Assuming renal function is normal, the patient's INs (fluid given to the animal) should closely match the OUTs (urinary output plus or minus vomitus, diarrhea, etc.) once hydration and volume status have been replenished. Urine output that does not meet the 1 to 2 mL/kg per hour minimum may be indicative of persistent hypovolemia. Inadequate urine output may also be due to fluid shifts such as third space losses or ongoing vomiting or diarrhea.

Monitoring urine output (volume) should be accompanied by measurement of specific gravity. Patients whose intravascular volume is depleted conserve volume by excreting less urine. The concentration of solids within the urine is high due to the low volume of urine. As a result, the USG is higher in these animals. An animal whose volume status is adequate or who has undergone volume resuscitation has little to no need to conserve volume and thus can excrete less concentrated urine. These patients pass urine with a lower USG.

Patients receiving fluid therapy often have a USG in the 1.020 to 1.030 range if renal function is adequate. A dehydrated patient whose renal function is adequate should have a USG greater than 1.030 (canine) and 1.035 (feline) (Mathews 2006d).

Chapter Summary

Monitoring hospitalized patients can be an extremely intensive process. Many parameters are recorded and evaluated throughout this practice. The job of patient monitoring is usually dedicated to the technician. The technician must evaluate each patient using his or her own powers of observation, regardless of how recently the patient has been evaluated by another party. Some aspects of patient monitoring are subjective, and as such, the technician will benefit from developing his or her own baseline interpretation of the patient's status. This baseline establishes a starting point from which the technician can easily observe a change in patient status.

Temperature should be measured a minimum of twice daily in hospitalized patients. Intermittent temperatures are most often monitored using a digital thermometer via rectal or axillary routes. More invasive methods of temperature measurement include continuous monitoring via rectal probe, core temperature measurement via thermistor, and infrared thermometry.

Normal temperature for cats and dogs falls between 37.5°C and 38.5°C. Temperatures outside this range warrant investigation. A patient is considered hypothermic if its temperature falls below 37.5°C. Warming may be achieved using blankets, oat bags, hot water bottles, circulating hot air blankets, or circulating hot water blankets. With use of any of these warming aids, it is imperative that the technician provide some type of buffer, such as a towel or blanket, between the patient and the warming aid. This is necessary to avoid the possibility of thermal burns.

Hyperthermia is not the same thing as pyrexia (fever). Hyperthermia is an increase in temperature caused by external sources. Pyrexia is a result of a condition affecting the patient's body from within. Patients that exhibit a body temperature greater than 39.5°C should be gently cooled. More invasive cooling measures are undertaken when temperatures reach 41°C and above.

HR and RR are monitored via several different routes. The most reliable sources of information are often the technician's powers of observation. Patient's that are monitored without a large degree of invasion often maintain resting HR and RRs that provide the technician with a truer sense of patient status. Intermittent or continuous ECGs or pulse oximetry are also helpful tools for monitoring HR and RR.

Body weight should be measured at least once a day in hospitalized animals. Sudden fluctuations in patient weight may be attributed to fluid gains or losses. One kilogram of body weight represents 1 L of fluid. The same scale should be used each time a weight is measured for a specific patient.

Central venous pressure measurement and blood pressure measurement are also valuable tools in the management of fluid therapy. Each may require advanced technical skills and can involve the use of expensive monitoring equipment. Noninvasive (indirect) blood pressure measurement is the most appropriate tool for the private practice setting because central venous catheterization and arterial catheterization are not required. Indirect blood pressure measurement can be accomplished using a Doppler system or an oscillometric monitor.

Measurement of urine output and USG yields information that is useful in tailoring fluid therapy. Volume of urine passed by a patient can be compared with the volume of fluid that the patient has received. It is helpful to know how much of the fluid therapy has remained with the patient. USG illustrates how concentrated the patient's urine is. In states of hypovolemia or dehydration, healthy kidneys conserve body water, which should cause an elevation in USG. Well-hydrated or diuresed patients have a lower USG.

Monitoring is a vital part of fluid therapy and largely the responsibility of the veterinary technician. It is necessary that the technician understand the importance of this role and ensure that every monitoring skill be used to its fullest extent.

Review Questions

1. Continuous temperature measurement can be achieved using a rectal probe. When might it be inappropriate to use this tool?
2. What is the difference between pyrexia and hyperthermia?
3. What is tachycardia?
4. Define bradycardia.
5. Identify two methods of measuring fluid gain or loss in a patient receiving fluid therapy in a hospital.
6. Weight gain or loss of 500 g over a short period of time represents a fluid gain or loss of approximately what volume?
7. CVP measurements that fall below the expected normal range may indicate which of the following conditions?
8. Elevated CVP measurements can indicate
9. Fluid therapy patients with normal renal function are expected to produce at least ___ ml/kg per hour of urine?

Answers to the review questions can be found on page 223 in the Appendix. The review questions are also available for download on a companion website at www.wiley.com/go/donohoenursing.

Further Reading

Craig, J., et al. 2000. Temperature measured at the axilla compared with rectum in children and young people: systematic review. *BMJ* 320:1174–1178.

Delaforcade, A., and E. Rozanski. 2001. Central venous pressure and arterial blood pressure measurements. *Vet Clin North Am* 31:1163–1174.

DiBartola, S., and S. Bateman. 2006. Introduction to fluid therapy. In *Fluid, Electrolyte, and Acid-Base Disorders in Small Animal Practice*, 325–344. St. Louis: Saunders.

Greer, R., et al. 2007. Comparison of three methods of temperature measurement in hypothermic, euthermic, and hyperthermic dogs. *JAVMA* 230:1841–1848.

Hammond, R., and C. Walters. 1999. Monitoring the Critical Patient. In *Manual of Canine and Feline Emergency and Critical Care*, 235–246. Cheltenham, UK: BSAVA.

Hansen, B. 2006. Technical aspects of fluid therapy. In S. DiBartola, ed. *Fluid, Electrolyte, and Acid-Base Disorders in Small Animal Practice*, 344–376. St. Louis: Saunders.

Kunkle, G., et al. 2004. Comparison of body temperature in cats using a veterinary infrared thermometer and a digital rectal thermometer. *JAAHA* 40:40–46.

Lagutchik, M. 2002. Fever in the ICU patient. In W. Wingfield, ed. *The Veterinary ICU Book*, 671–685. Jackson, WY: Teton NewMedia.

Mathews, K. 2006a. Accidental hypothermia. In *Veterinary Emergency and Critical Care Manual*. 291–296. Guelph, Ontario, Canada: LifeLearn.

Mathews, K. 2006b. Hyperthermia/Heatstroke/Malignant hyperthermia. In *Veterinary Emergency and Critical Care Manual*, 297–303. Guelph, Ontario, Canada: LifeLearn.

Mathews, K. 2006c. Management of acute renal failure. In *Veterinary Emergency and Critical Care Manual*, 709–722. Guelph, Ontario, Canada: LifeLearn.

Mathews, K. 2006d. Monitoring fluid therapy and complications of fluid therapy. In S. DiBartola, ed. *Fluid, Electrolyte, and Acid Base Disorders in Small Animal Practice*, 377–391. St. Louis: Saunders.

Mathews, K. 2006e. Sepsis/Septic shock. In *Veterinary Emergency and Critical Care Manual*, 588–596. Guelph, Ontario, Canada: LifeLearn.

Rudloff, E., and R. Kirby. 2001. Colloid and crystalloid resuscitation. *Vet Clin North Am* 31:1207–1230.

Spiess, B., and M. Gomez. 1998. Hemodynamic monitoring. In *Longnecker's Principles and Practice of Anesthesiology*, 802–828. St. Louis: Mosby.

Waddell, L. 2004. Blood pressure monitoring for the critically ill. Proceedings of Western Veterinary Conference.

Walters, J. M. 2002. Hyperthermia. In *The Veterinary ICU Book*, 1130–1136. Jackson, WY: Teton NewMedia.

Wingfield, W. 2002. Accidental hypothermia. In *The Veterinary ICU Book*, 1116-1129. Jackson, WY: Teton NewMedia.

Complications of Fluid Therapy

Complications associated with therapeutic administration of intravenous (IV) fluids do not occur with great frequency in veterinary patients. Those that do arise typically fall into one of two categories: catheter-associated complications and fluid-associated complications.

Catheter-Associated Complications

Fortunately, it is not extremely common to encounter problems associated with IV catheters. Many potential hazards can be avoided with proper care, preparation, and monitoring carried out by the veterinary technician.

As discussed in Chapter 3, appropriate use of catheters begins with selection of a catheter that is suitable for a particular patient. Use of short large-bore catheters is ideal for delivery of fluid boluses in patients that require rapid resuscitation. In contrast, patients receiving long-term IV therapy that involves the use of many different fluid types and compositions will be better served by centrally placed multilumen catheters. It is important to consider the health status of the patient before placement of an IV catheter because catheter type or location may be unsuitable due to the nature of the animal's illness. Hind limbs should not be selected for IV sites in patients experiencing diarrhea. In contrast, forelimbs are not the ideal choice for patients that are vomiting. Animals that would benefit from placement of a central line may not be ideal candidates due to coagulopathy or immune-mediated disease. All of these issues must be considered before placement in an attempt to reduce the potential for catheter-related complications. The nature of veterinary care is such that our patients may soil themselves in

Fluid Therapy for Veterinary Technicians and Nurses, First Edition. Charlotte Donohoe.
© 2012 Charlotte Donohoe. Published 2012 by John Wiley & Sons, Inc.

times of ill health. Such situations may lead to contamination of catheter sites and subsequent catheter-associated infection.

Vascular inflammation and infection

In addition to patient soiling and self-contamination, catheter sites that remain clean throughout the dwell time may develop infection as a result of improper preparation before placement (Burrows 1982). Human studies have shown that the most common bacterial isolates from infected catheter sites are organisms considered to be normal skin dwellers such as *Staphylococcus epidermidis* and *Staphylococcus aureus* (Marsh-Ng 2007). It is not uncommon to find growth of one of these organisms once the catheter is cultured. However, it *is* uncommon for the patient to develop septicemia as a result of this colonization (Tan 2003).

To reduce the chance of catheter contamination, the technician must prepare the catheter site in a way that minimizes the presence of normal skin flora. Catheter sites may be prepared in a variety of ways. The following are some guidelines that contribute to clean, safe placement of IV catheters.

- Clean area for procedure
  - Have supplies ready on clean surface
  - Have patient lying on clean surface
- Ensure a large clean field surrounding catheter site
  - Clip large area of fur
  - Using gauze squares soaked with surgical scrub, scrub entire area (3 to 5 minutes)
  - Using gauze squares soaked with alcohol, wipe area several times until square shows no debris
  - Using gauze squares soaked with tincture of chlorhexidine or iodine, wipe area several times ensuring no debris on gauze
- Use aseptic technique for placement of catheter
  - Catheter tip/proximal end of catheter should be only part of catheter that contacts patient
  - Dry, clean gauze square may be placed around limb to cover hair line to minimize any contact between catheter and skin or hair at periphery
- Ideally operator should wear gloves for any catheter placement; mandatory for placement of central lines
- An adhesive bandage with sterile pad (such as Band-Aid) can be placed over the point of insertion to maintain sterility
- Clean tape and bandage material will help sustain the clean environment of the catheter
- Sterile technique should be continued through connection of infusion set and fluid bag
- Lines should be kept off hospital floors whenever possible
- Fluid lines should be changed every 48 to 72 hours

IV catheters can become somewhat mobile within the vessel despite efforts to place them securely. Catheters may rotate slightly or move inward and outward. Any movement is detrimental to the health of the vessel within which the catheter is placed. Motion from the catheter causes irritation to the interior wall of the vessel. In addition, the in-and-out motion of the catheter can drag organisms from the skin into the vessel, another event that causes vessel irritation. *Phlebitis* is the term used to describe a blood vessel that is inflamed. An affected vessel typically appears slightly reddened and feels warm and somewhat hardened or ropy to the touch. If any of these symptoms are noted in a patient receiving IV therapy, it is necessary to remove the catheter and seek IV access elsewhere.

Phlebitis can also be caused by the type of fluid being infused. Solutions that contain glucose, amino acids, lipids, barbiturates, benzodiazepines, or chemotherapeutic agents all have a higher tendency to irritate the interior of the blood vessel (Maki 1991). Administration of parenteral nutrition is more safely achieved using a central line for this reason. The solutions used for parenteral nutrition are rich in amino acids and lipids and better tolerated by larger vessels.

Other factors affecting the development of phlebitis include catheter material, length of placement, catheter size and width, and patient health (Maki 1991).

Embolism

An embolus is a structure found within the vasculature (abnormal) that travels through a vessel and causes an obstruction. The term *embolus* does not specifically describe the nature of the structure causing the obstruction. It is possible for a patient to suffer from an air embolism or even a catheter embolism. A *thromboembolism* is a blood clot that can travel throughout the vasculature and cause an obstruction.

It is important to use extreme caution while removing an IV catheter because an accidental cut through the catheter can cause a catheter embolus. The technician should try to cut bandage material that is far from the catheter site. In addition, the catheter stylet should not be removed and replaced during placement because the stylet is likely to bore through the cannula and can also cause a catheter embolus in this manner.

A catheter embolus may be removed from a peripheral vessel if action is prompt. A tourniquet placed proximal to the catheter site will help reduce the chance of travel beyond the limb. A venous cut-down procedure may allow the clinician to locate and remove the catheter fragment (Spencer 1982).

An air embolism may accidentally be delivered to a veterinary patient receiving fluid therapy. Air bubbles in a solution set, an empty fluid bag, or administration of IV medication are but a few examples of where air emboli may originate. Small air emboli are most often clinically insignificant in veterinary patients. However, large or rapid IV boluses of air can cause cardiovascular collapse and shock (Tan 2003).

Intraosseous catheters

As with any type of catheter, infection is a possible cause of postoperative patient illness. Patients may suffer from osteomyelitis as a result of catheter contamination. Catheter position can also lead to complications in patients whose fluids are accidentally delivered extravascularly. This leads to cellulitis, a condition that can be painful to the patient. In some cases, improper placement of intraosseous (IO) catheters can damage the sciatic nerve (Moore 2006).

IO delivery of fluids at extremely high rates is thought to be painful to the patient. In addition, fluids that are cooler than room temperature also cause discomfort when delivered via IO catheters (Moore 2006).

Jugular catheters and central lines

Jugular catheters are excellent tools that facilitate many of the monitoring tasks undertaken by the veterinary technician. Although infrequent, problems do arise despite efforts to prevent them. Some difficulties are catheter specific; these were discussed in detail in Chapter 3. Other complications are associated with central lines or jugular catheters in general and are the focus of this discussion.

Thrombosis is of particular concern in many patients that warrant a jugular catheter. These patients are often critically ill and suffer from more than one condition. The potential for jugular vein thrombosis is increased in patients with immune-mediated disease, sepsis, or pancreatitis (Waddell 2002). Much consideration is needed to weigh the risks and the benefits associated with jugular catheter placement in these patients.

Patients with coagulation disorders are at high risk for developing complications with placement of central lines. It is not recommended to place these catheters in animals that have severe coagulopathies in the event that hemorrhage occurs and is not compressible. If the animal's coagulation capabilities are not severely diminished, it may be necessary to risk placement of a central line due to the severity of the animal's other clinical signs. Central lines should be placed in a location where compression of the vessel is possible. In the event that the catheter site undergoes some degree of bleeding, the technician should be able to manage the blood loss if the site is accessible. Placement of a jugular catheter is safer if carried out at a more cranial location rather than accessing the vessel farther down near the thoracic inlet.

Multilumen central lines may develop kinks at the site of insertion if the catheter hub and wings are not secured in line with the catheter. Difficulty obtaining blood samples is a relatively frequent occurrence with central lines. Some catheters sample with ease from one port and not at all from another. One can speculate this difficulty is related to catheter position and that it is possible for a port to butt against a valve or vessel wall, preventing the user from obtaining a blood sample.

Central lines often provide two or more separate lumens within the catheter. Patients can receive fluids through one lumen and have the additional port(s) available for sampling or administration of medications. These extra ports are usually maintained with a heparin lock, which is achieved by flushing the Luer adapter with heparinized saline at a concentration of 1 IU/mL. The flush is administered every 4 hours as well as after administration of medications or withdrawal of blood samples. The port is clamped after the flush, and the heparin helps prevent formation of a blood clot. In some cases, a blood clot forms within the lumen of an unused port and causes an obstruction. The technician is unable to flush the port if this occurs. Once the port is obstructed, it is no longer useful and can be labeled as such to save time. The catheter does not need to be removed or replaced if a superfluous port becomes obstructed. As long as the catheter provides adequate IV access and shows no signs of irritation, it can be left in place.

Suturing the catheter in place presents a challenge to the technician. Mild misdirection of the distal catheter and fluid lines may allow movement of the catheter. Sutures that are excessively tight will cause the patient discomfort. If the sutures are not snug enough, however, the catheter may move in and out of the patient's skin. This motion can lead to introduction of bacteria to the vessel resulting in a higher potential for infection (Spencer 1982).

Any movement of the catheter within the vessel also increases the risk of phlebitis. Because central lines are located in major vessels, the occurrence of phlebitis or thrombosis imparts more severe consequences when related to these catheters than with other peripherally placed cannulas. Jugular thrombosis, obstruction of the jugular vein by a blood clot, is a complication associated with jugular catheters. Patients with jugular thrombosis display a hardened ropy jugular vein that is sometimes warmer than normal to the touch. Obstruction of the jugular vein can lead to facial swelling (edema), nasal congestion, and dyspnea (Tan 2003).

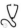 Nursing considerations

Daily evaluation of catheter bandages is a critical part of patient monitoring. Its importance should not be forgotten. Many patients present mildly or markedly dehydrated. It is at this juncture that catheter bandages are most often placed. Within several hours of initiation of fluid therapy, it is not uncommon to observe signs of swelling in the tissues proximal and distal to peripheral catheter bandages. In some instances, this swelling is not associated with infection but rather is evidence that a bandage suitable at time of placement is now too tight. Rehydration will lead to expansion of the intracellular space and tissues, and at times, bandage changes are needed to accommodate this expansion. Evaluation of the patient's toes and proximal limb is necessary to ensure the tissue is not expanding over the edges of the bandage.

Complications Associated with Fluid Choice

Selection of fluid type should be made with consideration given to an individual patient's specific needs. Illness causes a wide range of alterations in an animal's metabolic status and body fluid composition. Selection of a fluid that is inappropriate for a given patient can contribute to worsening of the condition and, in extreme cases, patient death.

Acidosis and alkalosis

An in-depth discussion of blood gases, acidosis, and alkalosis is beyond the scope of this text. However, to discuss arguments in favor of one fluid choice over another, it is necessary to have a basic awareness of these principles.

pH is the term used to describe the degree to which the blood is alkaline or acidic. Changes in pH are affected by hydrogen ions, carbon dioxide, bicarbonate (HCO_3), and electrolytes. Normal pH for canine and feline patients ranges between 7.35 and 7.45. Deviation below this range is representative of an acidemic state, whereas deviation above this range is representative of an alkalemic state. In sickness, animals often have a pH that departs from normal range. This departure can be the result of a primary cause or a combination of the primary cause and the body's reaction to this cause.

Several mechanisms within the body are responsible for maintaining balance between acids and bases. To simplify this discussion, the focus here is limited to the lungs and the kidneys.

Respiration contributes to the maintenance of proper pH by removing carbon dioxide, which is an acidifying component, from the animal's blood. Respiratory failure can lead to an increase in CO_2, leaving an increased acid component and thereby decreasing the pH of the animal's blood. The opposite is also true. If an animal has an increased respiratory rate, an increased amount of CO_2 is exchanged in the lungs and removed from

Table 7.1 Common Causes of Acid Base Disturbances

Metabolic acidosis	Diabetic ketoacidosis
	Ethylene glycol toxicity
	Sepsis
	Renal failure
	Poor perfusion
Metabolic alkalosis	Hypoxia
	Gastric vomiting
	Severe hypokalemia
	Pyloric obstruction
	Hyperadrenocorticism
Respiratory acidosis	Laryngeal paralysis
	Upper airway obstruction
	Heatstroke
	Neuromuscular diseases (tetanus, botulism, polyradiculoneuritis
	Pleural effusion
	Pneumonia
Respiratory alkalosis	Hyperventilation
	Heatstroke
	Pneumonia

the blood. In this case, a diminished acid component is left and the pH of the blood increases. This is an extreme simplification of this process. These two conditions are respectively named *respiratory acidosis* and *respiratory alkalosis*.

The kidneys also play a role in maintaining acid base balance. The lungs elicit changes in acid-base balance that are affected within minutes, whereas the kidneys elicit a slower change.

Bicarbonate is an ion found in the blood and represents the primary base component found in the plasma. Bicarbonate ions are conserved by the kidneys and returned to the blood depending on the hydrogen ion concentration. This is the main contribution of the kidneys to maintaining acid-base balance.

In times of illness, symptoms such as vomiting, diarrhea, fever, and anorexia can cause alterations in concentrations of various ions found in blood. Where blood gas analysis is available, it is prudent to evaluate a patient's acid-base balance before initiating fluid therapy.

Fluids used to treat veterinary patients are often categorized with respect to their acidifying or alkalinizing capacity. Much consideration is given to the patient's status before initiating fluid therapy so that the ill effects of administering an inappropriate solution are avoided. Table 7.1 summarizes the common causes of acid-base disturbances.

Fluid considerations

The fluid therapy prescription is not determined by the technician. It is the decision of the primary care clinician, and fluids are selected with specific goals in mind. The technician is often responsible for initiating the delivery of these fluids, and knowledge surrounding why specific selections are made can assist the technician in patient monitoring.

Crystalloid solutions are fluids frequently used in veterinary practice. Their constitution is mainly water mixed with sodium or glucose. These solutions are available with a variety of different electrolyte concentrations. Administration of crystalloids is appropriate in many clinical settings. These solutions equilibrate relatively soon after administration and redistribute throughout the interstitial and intracellular compartments. Different therapeutic goals may be achieved through the use of crystalloid solutions including replacement of fluid losses and provision of maintenance fluid needs.

Crystalloid solutions are categorized as either replacement solutions or maintenance solutions. Within these categories, fluids are further divided into acidifying solutions and alkalinizing solutions. Attention to these details contributes to appropriate fluid choices for patients receiving IV therapy.

Normal saline (0.9% NaCl) is an acidifying crystalloid solution. The pH of 0.9% NaCl is roughly 5.5; the same is true of LRS.

Alkalinizing solutions contain a component that is metabolized to HCO_3. LRS, Plasma-Lyte A, and Normosol R are examples of alkalinizing solutions.

Fluid selection is made with consideration to the pH of a solution, its acidifying/alkalinizing properties, its electrolyte composition, and its propensity for redistribution. Choice of an acidifying solution can be a great detriment to a patient suffering from metabolic acidosis. In contrast, using an alkalinizing solution such as LRS to treat a patient with severe liver disease is counterintuitive because the lactate within the solution is metabolized by the liver. LRS also contains calcium. As such, it is not a suitable fluid to pair with blood products and may not be an appropriate choice for a hypercalcemic patient.

Glucose-containing solutions are used with caution in veterinary patients. The glucose in the solution is metabolized by the body leaving free water to be redistributed to the body water compartments. This free water can lead to complications in patients that cannot tolerate the additional volume, such as patients suffering from heart failure.

Glucose-containing solutions also pose a greater risk than non-glucose-containing solutions where there is potential for extravascular administration. Extravasation of glucose solutions can lead to pain and swelling surrounding the catheter site.

Many patients that present to the veterinary hospital with severe illness are acidemic as a result of their disease. Alkalinizing solutions are frequently used at the onset of fluid therapy and help to restore appropriate acid-base balance. Plasma-Lyte A, Plasma-Lyte 148, and Normosol R are alkalinizing solutions. Acidifying solutions are used with less frequency, the most common being 0.9% sodium chloride (NaCl) (Mathews 1998). Although acidosis and alkalosis are not the only conditions treated by fluid therapy, it is good practice to consider acid-base balance when making fluid selections.

Colloids

Colloids are fluids that contain large particles. The size of these particles makes it difficult for the colloids to leave the vasculature. As the colloids stay within the vascular space, the large particles exert a force that attracts water; colloids succeed in maintaining or drawing water into the vasculature.

Both synthetic and natural colloids are used in veterinary patients. Plasma and fresh frozen plasma are natural colloids. They are blood products and as such require special storage protocols and may be challenging to obtain. However, their use in the critical care setting is common and beneficial to patients suffering from a variety of different conditions. Synthetic colloids are more easily stored and have less potential than natural colloids for causing an undesirable reaction in the patient.

Colloids help increase the intravascular volume by attracting water. Concurrent administration of colloids and crystalloids can quickly replenish the intravascular volume of a cardiovascularly compromised patient. The colloids also maintain the crystalloids within the vasculature for a longer period of time than they would normally remain.

As with any type of fluid administered to the veterinary patient, complications may arise if colloids are not used judiciously. Administration of colloids with crystalloids requires the volume of crystalloids to be reduced. Failing to reduce crystalloid volume may cause the pressure exerted by water molecules within the vasculature to exceed normal levels. This pressure is termed *intravascular hydrostatic pressure* and is the force exerted by water in an outward direction (leaving the vasculature). The intravascular hydrostatic pressure is increased due to the volume of crystalloids maintained in the vascular space. The increase in pressure leads to an increase in filtration at the level of the capillaries and subsequently to water shifting out of the vasculature and into the interstitium. Once in the interstitium the excess fluid leads to *interstitial edema*. Edema can be the result of overadministration of crystalloids in conjunction with colloids, but it can also be the result of overadministration of crystalloids alone.

The formation of edema within the interstitial space causes changes in cell structure within the tissues. Body water moves differently as a result, and pitting edema is the undesirable outcome. When the application of gentle pressure on a peripheral limb leaves an indent in the patient's skin that is slow to disappear, the patient has pitting edema.

Synthetic colloids have been reported to cause minor changes in coagulation times. To avoid serious complications associated with synthetic colloids, these products should be avoided in patients with preexisting coagulopathies (Mathews 2006a).

Overadministration of fluids

The science of fluid therapy is not exact. Upon presentation of emergency and critical care patients, the clinician puts forth his or her best effort in estimating the degree to which the animal is dehydrated or the volume of blood that has been lost. Every effort is made to replace the volume needed to restore the animal to health. In some cases, the volume delivered to the patient is overestimated and fluid therapy leads to overhydration. Effective monitoring reduces the chances of overhydration and alerts the medical team promptly if early signs of overhydration are detected. Patient monitoring can also help evaluate whether fluid therapy is yielding an appropriate response from the animal and help guide potential changes in the therapeutic plan.

Many clinical signs are associated with overadministration of fluids. Some of these signs are subtle, such as a slight increase in respiratory rate, pulmonary edema, patient restlessness, an increase in heart rate, or an increase in urine output. Other symptoms of fluid overload, such as chemosis, interstitial or peripheral edema, serous nasal discharge, and vomiting and diarrhea, are more obvious and rarely missed during patient evaluation.

Chemosis

Edematous patients may display conjunctiva that appear swollen and pronounced. The conjunctiva themselves are edematous, a condition that may arise with overadministration of fluids. This condition is referred to as *chemosis* and is one of the later signs of overadministration of fluids to appear (Mathews 2006b).

Serous nasal discharge

Many canine patients have a slight serous discharge from their nose on a regular basis. Appearance of new discharge or a noticeable increase from normal volume can indicate that the patient has received more fluids than it can manage. Close observation of any patient with serous nasal discharge is warranted.

Peripheral (interstitial) edema

Overadministration of fluids can cause an increase in the intravascular hydrostatic pressure. This increase in pressure results in larger volumes of fluid being filtered at the level of the capillaries. Subsequently, fluid shifts out of the intravascular compartment and moves into the interstitial space. The excess of fluid in the interstitial space is known as *interstitial edema* and is easily detected in a variety of locations on the animal. Recall that the technician can more easily distinguish between what is normal and what is edematous for a given patient if she or he has personally evaluated the patient before the onset of therapy.

The region surrounding the hock is an ideal area for assessment of edema. Because this area typically carries little excess tissue or fat, the inability to locate landmarks such as the lateral saphenous vein, the tendon located on the caudal aspect of the limb (Achilles tendon), or the beginning of the muscle bed cranial to the hock is attributed to the presence of interstitial edema.

Canine patients may develop edema around the lower portion of their head and neck, the area often referred to as jowls. In the edematous patient, this area becomes pendulous and quite mobile.

Pulmonary edema

Pulmonary edema is a serious complication associated with fluid therapy (Fig. 7.1). If the technician is not evaluating respiratory rate and ausculting lung sounds throughout patient treatment, it is possible to miss the signs associated with pulmonary edema because their onset may be subtle.

Fluid therapy causes an increase in the pressure caused by water within the pulmonary interstitium (hydrostatic pressure). As this occurs, fluid leaks from the interstitium into the alveoli causing pulmonary edema. Clinical signs encountered with pulmonary edema include an increased respiratory rate, productive cough with foamy and/or bloody sputum, decreased oxygen saturation, and tachycardia. Pulmonary edema is a risk for any patient receiving fluid therapy; however, animals that have diseases such as preexisting inflammatory conditions, pancreatitis, or sepsis are at greater risk for developing this complication (Mathews 2006b).

Pleural effusion

Pleural effusion is the abnormal accumulation of fluid within the pleural space (Figs. 7.2 and 7.3). Under normal circumstances, a small amount of fluid is present within the

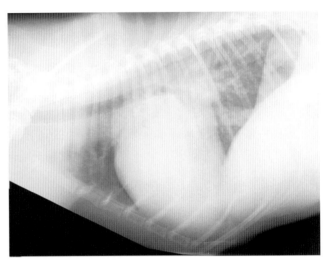

Figure 7.1. Lateral thoracic radiograph demonstrates pulmonary edema.

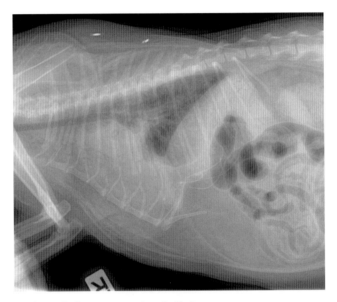

Figure 7.2. Thoracic radiograph demonstrates pleural effusion.

pleural space. Its function is to lubricate the surfaces of the visceral and parietal pleurae and reduce friction throughout the motions of respiration.

When excess fluid accumulates within this cavity, it occupies the potential space routinely used during respiration. It becomes increasingly difficult for the animal to expand its lungs to their fullest extent. The result is a respiratory pattern that is rapid and shallow. Oxygenation is compromised, and the patient experiences increasing levels of respiratory distress.

Common causes of pleural effusion are decreased oncotic pressure, increased intravascular hydrostatic pressure, and inflammatory processes. Overadministration of fluids contributes to an increase in hydrostatic pressure and can lead to pulmonary effusion if left untreated. In addition, a patient with pulmonary edema as a result of overhydration is also at risk for developing pleural effusion (Mathews 2006b). Fluid from the

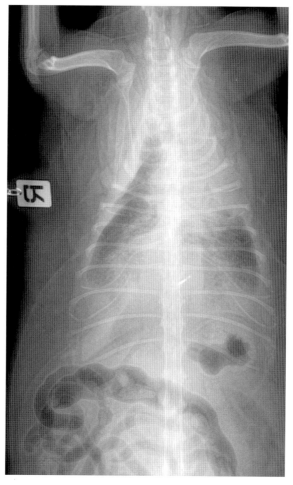

Figure 7.3. Thoracic radiograph demonstrates pleural effusion. Note the scalloped look of the right side of the lung outline due to the fluid surrounding the lungs.

pulmonary edema is able to shift across the pleural membrane (visceral pleura) and move into the pleural space causing it to become an effusion.

Chapter Summary

The potential for complications associated with fluid therapy is ever present. Awareness of this potential coupled with diligent patient monitoring contributes to a reduction in the risk of development of complications associated with fluid therapy.

When fluid therapy is initiated, consideration must be given to the health status of the patient, the purpose of the catheter placement, and the expectations for length of catheter dwell and fluid administration. Appropriate selection of catheter type and location plays an important role in the safety of fluid delivery.

Strict aseptic technique must be followed during placement of any catheter. Fluid administration sets, fluid bags, and fluid additives must be handled with the same degree of cleanliness because introduction of bacteria at any level is detrimental to patient health.

Securing and bandaging of catheters is an important role carried out by the technician. Catheter movement within the vessel can cause mild to marked damage to the vessel wall. Trauma to the vessel leads to inflammation within the vessel, also known as phlebitis. The occurrence of phlebitis is also influenced by other catheter characteristics. Catheter material, length, and bore size are also associated with an increased risk of phlebitis.

Thromboembolism, catheter embolism, and air embolisms involve the abnormal presence of each of these substances within the vessel. They are mobile within the vasculature and can cause severe complications.

Catheter bandages should be evaluated daily to ensure that patient rehydration has not led to swelling of the limb surrounding the bandage.

Central lines are extremely useful tools in critical care medicine. As with any other form of IV therapy, strict aseptic technique is mandatory during placement of central lines as well as during any form of handling throughout their use. Common complications associated with these catheters included kinks, blood clots within one or several lumens, and failure to sample. Placement of jugular catheters requires selection of a site that is easily compressible should bleeding exceed expectations during placement.

Movement of the catheter within the jugular vein can lead to inflammation and obstruction of the vessel. Venous obstruction at this location is accompanied by clinical signs such as facial swelling/edema, nasal congestion, and possibly dyspnea.

Fluid selection is an important part of therapy and can be associated with a variety of complications. Fluids should be chosen with the goal of selecting a fluid type that is appropriate for each individual patient. Electrolyte content, pH, rate of redistribution, and goals of therapy (replacement vs. maintenance) are all characteristics that should be considered during fluid choice. Selection of inappropriate fluids can lead to a deterioration of the patient's condition.

Overadministration of fluid therapy is an unfortunate complication of fluid therapy. Despite the efforts of the medical team, hydration estimates can be overzealous, and latent preexisting conditions can remain undetected in newly admitted patients. Overadministration of fluids can lead to the clinical signs listed in Table 7.2. Note that individual patients may display one or several of these clinical signs. Investigation of even the slightest change is warranted to allow prompt treatment of fluid overload.

Table 7.2   Clinical Signs Associated with Fluid Overload

- Increased respiratory rate
- Restlessness
- Coughing
- Peripheral edema
- Pulmonary edema
- Chemosis
- Serous nasal discharge
- Vomiting
- Diarrhea
- Pleural effusion

Review Questions

1. Phlebitis refers to
   a. A skin irritation cause by clippers
   b. Excessive bleeding from the catheter site
   c. Normal skin flora
   d. Inflammation of a blood vessel
2. A thromboembolism is a _____ that can cause an obstruction anywhere in the vasculature.
3. Central lines may be contraindicated in which of the following patients?
   a. Patients with diabetes
   b. Patients with airway disease
   c. Coagulopathic patients
   d. Anemic patients
4. List three possible clinical signs associated with overadministration of fluids.
5. Assessing the area surrounding a patient's hock is helpful in identifying which complication associated with fluid therapy?

Answers to the review questions can be found on page 224 in the Appendix. The review questions are also available for download on a companion website at www.wiley.com/ go/donohoenursing.

Further Reading

Burrows, C. 1982. Inadequate skin preparation as a cause of intravenous catheter-related infection in the dog. *J Am Vet Med Assoc* 180:747–749.

Hughes, D., & A. Boag. 2006. Fluid therapy with macromolecular plasma volume expanders. In S. DiBartola, ed. *Fluid, Electrolyte, and Acid-Base Disorders in Small Animal Practice*, 621–634. St. Louis: Saunders.

Maki, D., and M. Ringer. 1991. Risk factors for infusion-related phlebitis with small peripheral venous catheters. *Ann Intern Med.* 114:845–854.

Marsh-Ng, M., D. Burney, and J. Garcia. 2007. Surveillance of infections associated with intravenous catheters in dogs and cats in an ICU. *J Am Anim Hosp Assoc* 43:13–20.

Mathews, K. 1998. The various types of parenteral fluids and their indications. *Vet Clin North Am* 28:483–513.

Mathews, K. 2006a. Fluid therapy: non-hemorrhage. In *Veterinary Emergency and Critical Care Manual*, 347–372. Guelph, Ontario, Canada: LifeLearn.

Mathews, K. 2006b. Monitoring fluid therapy and complications of fluid therapy. In S. DiBartola, ed. *Fluid, Electrolyte, and Acid-Base Disorders in Small Animal Practice*, 377–391. St. Louis: Saunders.

Mazzaferro, E. 2008. Complications of fluid therapy. *Vet Clin Small Anim Pract* 38:607–619.

Rudloff, E., and R. Kirby. 2009. Fluid resuscitation and the trauma patient. *Vet Clin North Am* 38:645–652.

Spencer, K. 1982. Intravenous catheters. *Vet Clin North Am Small Anim Pract* 12:533–543.

Tan, R., A. Dart, and B. Dowling. 2003. Catheters: a review of the selection, utilization and complications of catheters for peripheral venous access. *Aust Vet J* 81:136–139.

Waddell, L. 2002. Advanced vascular access options. Proceedings of American College of Veterinary Internal Medicine Conference.

Fluid Types

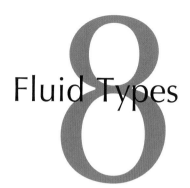

Choosing a suitable fluid type for intravenous (IV) therapy is a task that deserves much thought. The needs of individual patients differ, and there is not one single fluid type suitable for all veterinary patients. Selection of appropriate fluids is the responsibility of the attending clinician. However, it is prudent for the technician to have a basic understanding of the differences in the fluids available for therapeutic use.

Fluids are divided into the categories of crystalloids and colloids. The colloids can be further divided into synthetic colloids and natural colloids.

Crystalloids

Crystalloids are the most commonly used type of fluid in veterinary practice. These solutions contain varying degrees of sugar or salt. They consist of relatively small low molecular weight particles and as such are not restricted in their movement throughout body water compartments.

Recall that oncotic pressure is the force exerted by proteins within the vasculature that draw water from the extravascular space into the vascular space. Osmotic pressure is the pressure generated by the contents of the interstitium and applies a force from the interstitium into the blood vessel. Finally, hydrostatic pressure is the force exerted by particles within the vasculature that push out of the vessel.

Crystalloids do not contribute to oncotic pressure, but they *do* contribute to osmotic pressure. This is partially due to the fact that crystalloid administration has its most noticeable effects in the interstitial space. Crystalloids that are delivered IV do not remain in the intravascular space indefinitely. Rather, they cross the vascular membrane

Fluid Therapy for Veterinary Technicians and Nurses, First Edition. Charlotte Donohoe.
© 2012 Charlotte Donohoe. Published 2012 by John Wiley & Sons, Inc.

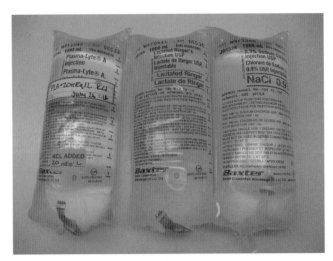

Figure 8.1. Plasma-Lyte A, lactated Ringer solution, and 0.9% sodium chloride are common selections for replacement solutions.

and enter the interstitial compartment. This happens relatively quickly; within approximately 1 to 2 hours of administration (Rudloff 2001). By this time, most of the crystalloids have left the intravascular space. It is estimated that 1 hour after IV delivery of crystalloids, only 20%–25% of the volume administered remains within the vasculature (Silverstein 2009).

Replacement crystalloids

Crystalloid fluids can be subdivided into the categories of maintenance solution or replacement solution. Replacement solutions are the first choice of crystalloids for patients that present to the hospital with clinical signs of dehydration (Fig. 8.1). These fluids are isotonic and have a sodium concentration similar to that of the extracellular fluid.

Replacement crystalloid solutions also contain components that affect the pH of body water. Acetate and lactate are two examples of buffers found in replacement crystalloid solutions. Lactate is metabolized by the patient's liver to form bicarbonate. Bicarbonate's influence raises the pH of the blood. The presence of buffers makes Plasma-Lyte A (PLA), Normosol R, and lactated Ringer solution (LRS) excellent choices for intravascular volume support in emergency and critical care patients. The buffers found in these replacement fluids contribute to the fluids' alkalinizing capability. The pH range for PLA, Normosol R, and LRS is from 6.5 to 7.4 (Mathews 2006a). These fluids also contain electrolytes, which are important considerations for patients needing volume resuscitation. Electrolytes are lost in varying quantities depending on the nature of the illness affecting the patient. On the contrary, some diseases cause elevations in certain electrolytes, another important consideration during fluid selection because the clinician may wish to avoid increasing an already elevated electrolyte value.

Normal saline (0.9% NaCl) is also a replacement solution but does not contain any buffers or electrolytes other than sodium and chloride. The absence of buffers means that 0.9% NaCl is considered an acidifying solution (Moore 2003). The pH of 0.9%

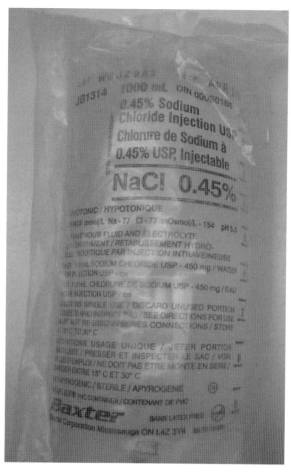

Figure 8.2. This 0.45% sodium chloride is an example of a maintenance solution.

NaCl is 5.0. Normal saline is often the fluid of choice in patients with hyponatremia or in patients whose profuse vomiting has led to a metabolic alkalosis. Animals suffering from a pyloric obstruction often present to the hospital with a profound hypochloremia. In this instance, 0.9% NaCl may be the replacement crystalloid of choice to reestablish appropriate chloride levels (Metheny 1992).

Maintenance crystalloids

Maintenance crystalloids contain less sodium than replacement fluids (Fig. 8.2). The concentration of sodium is approximately half that of the plasma (Rudloff 2001). Hospitalized animals often fail to consume an adequate volume of water via eating or drinking to maintain their hydration and overall volume of body water. After establishing that the patient's hydration and vascular volume are within normal limits, it is often necessary to maintain this status via continued fluid therapy. Maintenance fluids are primarily used in hospitalized animals to prevent loss of body water and electrolytes when the animal is not inclined to maintain these on their own. It is not uncommon for replacement crystalloids to be used for maintenance of hydration status in patients whose illness causes ongoing losses in excess of those associated with normal metabolic function.

Approximately an hour after IV administration, ~10% of maintenance crystalloids remain within the vasculature. For this reason, maintenance crystalloids are rarely used for replacement of intravascular volume. They are most often given at a slower rate with a goal of replenishing the extravascular spaces. The primary reason for using maintenance crystalloids is that the fluids equilibrate throughout the body water compartments, partially replenishing the intravascular and interstitial spaces, and more adequately replenishing the intracellular space. As such, these fluids are indicated in patients that are not suffering from severe ongoing daily losses but rather cannot maintain their body water balance via normal means.

Maintenance crystalloids are characterized by a low sodium concentration and a low chloride concentration. These fluids also contain potassium and in some examples contain dextrose as well. Maintenance fluids are hypotonic, whereas replacement fluids are isotonic. For this reason, maintenance fluids should not be administered at extremely high rates over short periods of time (as a bolus). Bolus administration of maintenance crystalloids can lead to complications such as cerebral edema (Silverstein 2009).

Examples of maintenance crystalloid solutions are 0.45% NaCl, Normosol M, and Plasmalyte 56.

Hypertonic saline

Hypertonic saline (HTS) is a crystalloid solution used for rapid volume expansion (Fig. 8.3). The term *hypertonic* refers to the fact that its concentration of sodium and chloride is greater than that of normal saline (0.9% NaCl). This also means that its concentrations of Na^+ and Cl^- are greater than that of plasma.

HTS replenishes the intravascular space by drawing body water from the interstitium and intracellular space into the vasculature. In so doing, the vascular space is quickly replenished and fluid is held within the space by the hypertonicity of the solution for a short time. The numerous sodium particles eventually diffuse out of the vascular space,

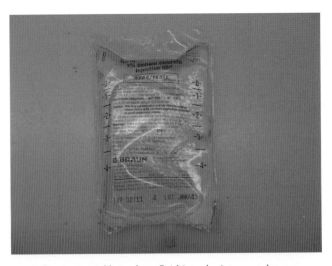

Figure 8.3. Hypertonic saline acts quickly to draw fluid into the intravascular space.

and the hypertonic effects of the HTS cease to exist. The diffusion of sodium out of the vasculature occurs approximately 30 minutes after infusion, and as such, the effects of HTS are short lived.

HTS is an excellent fluid choice for the treatment of severe hypovolemic shock; however, its use must be carried out with caution. HTS is not appropriate for use in patients that are severely dehydrated. These patients do not have adequate body water stores in their intracellular and interstitial spaces to permit fluid to shift safely out of these compartments. To avoid causing intracellular dehydration, it is advisable to administer HTS and follow administration with a crystalloid solution to maintain the body water volume in the interstitial and intracellular compartments.

Patients with cardiac disease are also at increased risk of complications if HTS is used during their therapy. An animal whose heart is not functioning at a normal healthy capacity is unlikely to be able to tolerate the rapid increase in intravascular volume associated with the administration of HTS.

HTS should not be used in patients that are hypernatremic or at high risk for developing hypernatremia. Because the infusion itself raises serum sodium levels, it is of particular danger in patients already manifesting this condition.

With illness involving uncontrolled hemorrhage, there is much debate regarding the benefits of HTS. Studies have shown that low-volume resuscitation is associated with positive outcome in patients suffering from severe trauma and hemorrhage. In addition, it appears that the use of hypertonic saline is an appropriate way to achieve low-volume resuscitation and that the benefits of its use are plentiful.

When compared with LRS, the volume of HTS required to augment intravascular volume is much smaller, meaning that infusion times are shorter (Mensack 2008). HTS has also demonstrated a protective relationship with red blood cells. In trauma patients, various factors combine to cause red blood cells (RBCs) to become less flexible than normal. When these cells lose their flexibility, they also lose the ability to pass through semipermeable membranes with their normal ease. HTS has been shown to contribute to the maintenance of RBC flexibility, a trait associated with more positive outcomes postresuscitation (Homma et al. 2005).

HTS has also been reported to protect against acute lung injury, contribute to a decrease in acute gut injury, avoid activation of inflammatory processes, and decrease intracranial pressure (Homma et al. 2005; Sheikh et al. 1996).

 ## *Nursing considerations*

Administration of hypertonic saline solution requires continuous monitoring and nursing care. Blood pressure, heart rate, and electrocardiogram should be monitored throughout administration. Extremely rapid infusion of HTS may cause hypotension and bradycardia (Mensack 2008). Judicious use of this crystalloid fluid improves its safety.

Colloids

In contrast to crystalloid fluids, colloids are fluids that contain large molecular weight particles. When administered into the intravascular space colloids remain, whereas crystalloids eventually move into other compartments. This is because the colloid molecules are larger in size than the healthy capillary pores. An exception to this rule occurs when a patient's endothelium is compromised and its capillaries develop leaks (e.g., during sepsis, severe trauma, or burn injuries). An additional difference between crystalloids and colloids is that colloids contribute to oncotic pressure, whereas crystalloids do not (Bateman 2003). As such, colloids offer far greater vascular volume expansion per volume administered than crystalloids do.

In health, colloids delivered into the vasculature not only hold fluid within this space, but they also draw fluid from other compartments. Patients suffering from loss of body water from the interstitial and intracellular compartments will be further compromised by the fluid shift caused by colloid administration. For this reason, crystalloids should be administered alongside colloids. Adjunctive crystalloid administration will help with volume expansion of the intravascular space but will also replenish the extravascular spaces.

The primary effect of colloids is exerted on the intravascular space, and colloids do not act to replenish the extravascular compartments. Administration of crystalloids in addition to colloids is recommended for protection of the interstitial and intracellular compartments.

Colloid administration requires continuous, diligent monitoring. Negative side effects associated with colloid administration include anaphylactoid reactions, volume overload, and in some cases vomiting and hypotension. Colloids must be used with caution in animals with cardiac disease or renal compromise because vascular volume expansion is not well tolerated in these patients.

Synthetic colloids

Colloids are divided into the categories of synthetic and natural. Synthetic colloids are composed of gelatins, dextrans, and hydroxyethyl starches. Some examples of synthetic colloids are dextran 40, dextran 70, hetastarch, pentastarch, and Oxyglobin (Fig. 8.4).

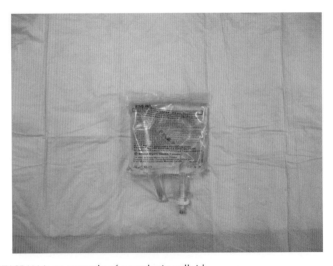

Figure 8.4. PENTASPAN is an example of a synthetic colloid.

Hetastarch

Hetastarch particles have a molecular weight that exceeds dextrans. These large particles remain in the patient's plasma for ~36 hours. Negative side effects of hetastarch administration are minimal but do exist. Some animals have been reported to experience allergic reactions post administration of hetastarch (Center 2006). Rapid bolus administration may cause histamine release in feline patients. This reaction is avoidable in most cases if the hetastarch administration is achieved over a period of 15 to 20 minutes. Patients receiving doses in excess of normal may experience some degree of compromise in coagulation. This compromise has not been associated with spontaneous or clinically significant bleeding.

Dextrans

Dextran 40 and dextran 70 contain large molecular weight particles compared with crystalloids but smaller than those found in hetastarch. In situations requiring rapid vascular volume expansion, dextran 70 is the more popular choice of the two. This is because its particles (molecular weight of 70 Da) exert a greater attractive force on body water than those contained in dextran 40 (40 Da).

Dextrans have a shorter life in the patient's plasma than hetastarch molecules. An additional drawback to these products is that they interact with RBCs in such a way that difficulty may arise with future cross matches of the patient's blood. If it is likely that the patient may need transfusion of blood products throughout its therapy, it is advisable to draw blood for typing before administration of Dextran solutions. Dextrans also interact with platelets, causing minor prolongation of coagulation times (Bateman 2003). Similar to hetastarch, anaphylactic reactions may arise with the use of dextrans (Center 2006).

Pentastarch

One of the primary advantages to pentastarch is its association with fewer effects on coagulation than the other synthetic colloids. It has the same beneficial effects as hetastarch, interferes less with platelet function, and is eliminated more quickly. After 24 hours, only 10% of the total volume infused remains in the patient's plasma. As with the other synthetic colloids, its use is not recommended in patients with cardiac or renal compromise. These patients are unable to manage the sudden increase in intravascular volume.

Oxyglobin

Oxyglobin falls into the subcategory of hemoglobin-based oxygen-carrying fluids. Oxyglobin is a sterile solution for IV use. It is a hemoglobin-based product carried in a balanced solution of salt. Its primary use is for the treatment of anemia. Oxyglobin exerts effects similar to the other synthetic colloids in terms of vascular volume replacement. It also provides additional oxygen-carrying capacity through its increased concentration of hemoglobin. Its administration effectively expands plasma volume. In some cases, its capacity to expand plasma volume may be more effective than anticipated, leading to volume overload (Bateman 2003). Oxyglobin also causes vasoconstriction and can cause increases in blood pressure. Extreme care during selection of volume and rate for IV delivery of this product increase its margin of safety.

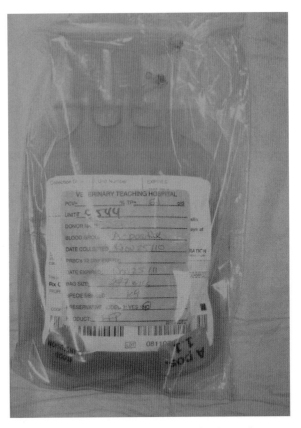

Figure 8.5. Fresh frozen plasma is a natural colloid. It is helpful to know the recipient's blood type before administration of any blood product.

Because Oxyglobin contains no RBCs, it is not necessary to perform any type of cross match before its administration. An additional benefit to this product is that it may be stored at room temperature and has a fairly lengthy shelf life (3 years).

A disadvantage of Oxyglobin is that once it has been administered, it is difficult to interpret various laboratory results for the recipient. Medical personnel may notice a discoloration of the patient's skin, urine, mucous membranes, and/or sclera with use of this product. None of these changes have been reported to be permanent. Oxyglobin remains in the patient's circulation for approximately 24 hours.

Negative side effects associated with the use of Oxyglobin include vomiting and melena, but these complications are rare. At time of print, Oxyglobin is unavailable.

Natural colloids and blood products

Natural colloids are high molecular weight solutions derived from species-specific donors. These include frozen or stored plasma (SP), fresh frozen plasma (FFP), whole blood (WB), and human serum albumin (HSA), which is available in different concentrations (Fig. 8.5). Natural colloids have a similar effect to synthetic colloids in that they increase intravascular volume and exert more lasting effects on this compartment than crystalloid fluids. In addition, natural colloids such as fresh WB and FFP contain clotting factors that may be beneficial to patients whose coagulation abilities are compromised. In resuscitation situations, the use of colloids can provide quicker volume support because smaller volumes achieve similar effects to large volume crystalloid administration. Natural colloids are particularly useful in resuscitation efforts in patients that have suffered massive trauma and significant loss of blood volume.

A number of drawbacks are associated with the use of natural colloids, but these are far outweighed by the benefits. Caution should be exercised using any of the natural colloids because they are all components of species specific blood. As such, it is possible for patients to experience anaphylactoid reactions during or after administration.

Fresh frozen plasma

FFP is obtained by separating components of WB. Once blood has been collected, plasma may be separated from the cellular portion by centrifugation. The blood is centrifuged at high speed, and the plasma is withdrawn and stored separately. If the plasma is separated and frozen within 6 hours of collection, it is considered FFP (Brooks 2003). FFP is stored at very low temperatures (−20°C) for up to 1 year.

FFP is often used in patients with coagulopathies. It may be used in animals with anticoagulant rodenticide toxicity, vitamin K deficiency, hepatic disease, von Willebrand factor deficiency, or disseminated intravascular coagulation. In recent years, FFP has been a popular component of treatment for pancreatitis. Despite this trend, it has yet to be proven that FFP is beneficial for these patients.

Although FFP contains a significant amount of proteins, it is not the most effective way to raise protein levels in a hypoproteinemic patient.

Albumin is one of the most important proteins found in plasma. It represents 50% of total plasma protein and generates most of the plasma's oncotic pressure (Trow et al. 2008). Decreased plasma protein levels can have considerable side effects in patients already compromised by illness.

FFP may be used as an initial means of diminishing the negative side effects of hypoproteinemia, but the volume required to raise protein levels significantly renders it an inefficient method of treating this condition. Canine plasma contains 25 to 30 g of albumin per liter (Cohn et al. 2007). To improve albumin concentration in hypoalbuminemic patients, it is recommended to administer 6 to 10 mL/kg FFP every 8 hours. This is thought to raise albumin levels by 0.5 g/dL (Logan et al. 2001). In a 25-kg canine patient, this would require administration of 250 mL FFP three times daily. Although FFP is effective at decreasing the side effects of hypoproteinemia, such as peripheral edema, it is a costly means of doing so. In addition, administration of such large volumes of FFP may exhaust available supplies and may also pose a risk of volume overload to the respective patient. Commercially available natural colloids, such as human serum albumin, may be a more appropriate choice than FFP for treatment of hypoproteinemia.

Stored plasma

Stored plasma (SP) is a natural colloid obtained by separating whole blood via centrifugation. In contrast to FFP, SP is not required to be separated and frozen within 6 hours of collection. The main difference between FFP and SP is the absence of coagulation factors in SP. SP still contains albumin and globulin, but it does not contain clotting factors V & VIII, important coagulation components that *are* present in FFP. FFP is relabeled as SP if it is stored beyond the 1-year mark. With lengthy storage, coagulation factors lose their potency, and the plasma is no longer useful for its hemostatic effects. SP can be frozen at −18°C for up to 5 years (Wardrop 2004).

Stored plasma is useful in several situations where coagulation factors are not required. Patients with severely decreased protein levels (i.e., <4.0 g/dL) benefit from treatment with SP (Mathews 2008). With severe protein loss, fluid is able to leak out of the vasculature and lead to interstitial edema. Administration of SP supports oncotic pressure and draws fluid into the intravascular space. Patients with marked hypoalbuminemia can also benefit from administration of SP for similar reasons. Animals with leaky capillaries are less likely to develop edema with administration of SP. However, this product must be used with caution because compromised capillaries may also leak large protein particles and lead to more severe edema. If large proteins leak out of the vascular space, they still have the capacity to attract water but will do so in the interstitium. Further accumulation of water in the interstitium further contributes to the formation of edema.

Stored plasma may also be used in conjunction with other blood products. For example, in animals suffering from whole blood loss, SP may be administered in conjunction with packed red blood cells (PRBCs) to replenish blood volume. This may be the only option in clinics where WB is not available. Where SP and PRBCs are available from different donors, test doses must be administered for each product to determine which product, if any, has triggered an adverse reaction in the patient.

Human serum albumin

Human serum albumin (HSA) is a colloidal solution suitable for IV administration in canine veterinary patients. It is derived from human blood obtained from donors in registered blood donor programs. The serum is separated from the blood cells and undergoes a rigorous sterilization process. Donors are required to participate in a screening process within 2 months of their donation. Screening tests include but are not limited to illnesses such as hepatitis B, hepatitis C, and human immunodeficiency virus. Despite the precautions used during collection of human serum, it is advisable for veterinary staff to use gloves when handling HSA or preparing for patient administration.

After the serum is sterilized and bottled, it takes on a pale yellow tinge and remains transparent. It contains approximately 96% albumin (Mazzaferro et al. 2002). HSA is a natural colloid, and its particles are larger than those contained in crystalloid solutions. In addition, the HSA particles are quite uniform, with similar weights and sizes. The solution is highly water soluble, and its particles carry a negative charge (Martin 2004). HSA does not contain clotting factors.

HSA is packaged in bottles and available in quantities of 50, 100, 250, or 500 mL. These volumes are available in different concentrations: 25% for the two smallest volumes or 5% for the two largest volumes.

The 5% solution contributes an oncotic pressure similar to that of plasma. As such, it is considered isoncotic and remains in the intravascular space without causing tremendous intercompartmental fluid shifts. The 25% solution is considered hypertonic to the plasma and generates an oncotic pull that exceeds that in the normal intravascular space. The hypertonicity creates an exaggerated pull and draws body water into the vasculature. One of the benefits encountered with use of the higher concentration of HSA is that a small volume of this solution generates a large effect. Opinions differ slightly, but it is generally accepted that administration of 25% HSA draws a volume of body water between three and five times the volume of HSA administered into the vascular space (Cohn 2007; Martin 2004). So administration of 100 mL of 25% solution generally augments the intravascular volume by approximately 400 mL within ~1 hour of administration.

As with any blood product, benefits and drawbacks are associated with administration of HSA. One of the major benefits of HSA is that it has a relatively long shelf life; storage requires no special equipment or refrigeration. The bottles can be stored for up to 3 years at room temperature. Once the bottle has been spiked for use, it should be used within 4 hours. The solution remaining in the bottle after 4 hours should be discarded. To facilitate delivery, different concentrations of HSA may be generated by sterile combination of HSA with 0.9% NaCl or 5% dextrose solutions. Sterile delivery from the HSA bottle is achieved through use of a vented solution set. Because the bottle is unable to collapse as the solution leaves, a vent is required to relieve the vacuum or negative pressure that develops within the bottle. A needle through the rubber stopper is an unsuitable solution because there is no barrier preventing environmental contaminants from entering the bottle through the needle hub. Vented solution sets include a filter that maintains sterility by blocking microparticles from entering the solution via the vent.

Few drawbacks are associated with the actual product of HSA; however, there are important clinically relevant drawbacks associated with its administration to the veterinary patient. With respect to the product itself, the main disadvantage is the associated cost. Cost varies depending on the country of purchase and the product manufacturer selected, but it is consistently higher than that associated with other natural colloids.

Drawbacks associated with administration generally involve adverse reactions from respective patients. It is important to remember that HSA is a product derived from a different species, and as such, it is essentially a foreign protein being introduced into the patient's vascular space. Administration of HSA may lead to side effects such as hypothermia, hypotension, vomiting, diarrhea, urticaria, and facial swelling. Hypocalcemia is a complication also associated with HSA administration caused by the increased level of albumin suddenly available in circulation. Free calcium binds to albumin; with more albumin available, there is an increase in the frequency of this reaction. The result is a decrease in ionized calcium.

There is no way to predict which patients will have severe reactions to HSA, making continuous monitoring mandatory during infusion. Patients may show signs of anaphylaxis after receiving extremely small volumes of HSA (Cohn 2007). In addition, it is generally recommended not to administer additional HSA transfusions more than 7 days after the initial infusion because the patient may develop product specific antigens, predisposing to more severe reactions (Trow et al. 2008). However, a 2005 study included two patients that received multiple HSA transfusions months apart with no adverse reactions (Mathews and Barry 2005).

To decrease the potential for adverse patient reactions, it is advisable to deliver a test dose of HSA before administration at full transfusion rate. Test doses allow the technician to monitor the initial reaction of the patient after only a small volume has been administered at a relatively slow infusion rate. The technician should perform and record a patient temperature, pulse, respiration (TPR) before starting the test. Once this is accomplished, the HSA may be delivered via infusion pump at a *rate* of 0.25 mL/kg per hour. This rate is delivered for 15 minutes and then a TPR is repeated. Any significant changes in any of the measured parameters should be investigated, and the clinician should be promptly notified. In my experience, it is most common to measure elevations in the TPR parameters, but the opposite is also possible. If there is any uncertainty with respect to whether or not the patient is in the early stages of a transfusion reaction, the test dose may be repeated and the patient's vitals measured once again. If there are further changes to the patient's vitals, the clinician may choose to treat the patient with antihistamines and continue the transfusion or discontinue the transfusion permanently and find an alternative product.

Despite all precautions, it is also possible that the patient experience a delayed transfusion reaction. There may be no noticeable change in patient vitals, comfort level, or demeanor during the transfusion. Reactions have been reported up to 7 days posttransfusion of HSA. These tend to include urticaria, facial edema, and pruritus (Cohn 2007).

In spite of the potential for adverse reaction to HSA, the usefulness of this solution renders it an obvious choice in specific clinical situations. Indications for HSA transfusion generally involve hypoalbuminemia or clinical signs related to illness that affects functions strongly associated with a patient's albumin concentration.

Albumin plays many important roles in a healthy animal. Approximately 40% of an animal's total body albumin is found within the vascular space (Mathews 2008). It is responsible for 80% of oncotic pressure (Trow et al. 2008). Albumin is partially responsible for maintenance of intravascular volume. At normal levels, it reduces microvascular permeability and in so doing, contributes to maintenance of normal albumin concentration through prevention of albumin loss. Albumin is also responsible for binding different substances within the circulatory system. It transports drugs, metabolites, and electrolytes and plays a significant role in maintaining fluid balance. Hypoalbuminemia is often associated with generalized edema and ascites.

Patients with refractory hypotension, severe hypoalbuminemia, peritonitis, or hypovolemia may be candidates for HSA transfusion. It is often the solution of choice when other colloidal infusions have failed to reverse clinical signs.

HSA transfusion is not used to treat conditions involving hypoxia or coagulopathies because it does not offer oxygen-carrying capacity, platelets, or clotting factors. This solution is not appropriate for patients that are severely dehydrated, experiencing cardiac insufficiency or failure, or those that are anemic.

It is reported that coagulation times may increase in human patients after administration of HSA. This is mainly due to a decrease in platelet count and the dilution of clotting factors associated with the increase in intravascular volume (Martin 2004).

Whole blood

The term *whole blood* is entirely descriptive of the contents of this fluid type. It is blood that has been collected from the intravascular compartment of a donor animal and mixed with an appropriate volume of anticoagulant plus or minus cell nutrient. The blood is not centrifuged, separated, or frozen before administration to a recipient. It is refrigerated during storage and should be maintained at a temperature between 1°C and 6°C (Fig. 8.6).

WB is delivered to the recipient via a blood transfusion administration set, which has a filter with pores that measure 170 μm in size (Green 2002). The filter is required to remove any clumps or blood clots that may have formed during the collection.

WB stored in citrate-phosphate-dextrose-adenine (CPDA)-1 is safely stored for up to 28 days. Depending on the condition of the recipient and the reason for transfusion, it may be preferable to administer WB that has been stored for a short period of time. For example, a patient that is anemic due to hemolysis will benefit from WB that is less than 5 days old (Green 2002). As blood is stored, the RBCs become less viable as they

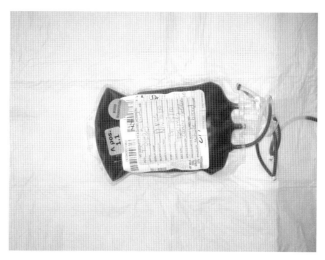

Figure 8.6. One unit of canine whole blood is approximately 450 mL.

age. Older RBCs are more fragile and thus more susceptible to destruction via hemolysis. In contrast, an anemic patient whose blood volume is depleted due to hemorrhage, with no evidence of coagulopathy, can benefit from fresh WB or blood that has been stored for more than 5 days.

Stored WB contains levels of ammonia that increase in direct relation to the length of storage. Patients with hepatic encephalopathy or elevated levels of ammonia should receive WB that is less than 5 days old if transfusion is necessary (Mathews 2006a).

WB is the fluid of choice for patients suffering from rapid loss of RBCs and plasma (WB). This loss is commonly seen in cases of trauma and anticoagulant rodenticide toxicity. Severe hemorrhage may occur during some types of surgery; WB is indicated in this situation as well.

Packed cell volume can also be used as a guideline for WB transfusion. Canine patients with a packed cell volume (PCV) less than 25% and feline patients with a PCV less than 20% are candidates for WB transfusion (Mathews 2006b). If there is a coagulopathy present in addition to the anemia, it is most beneficial to transfuse fresh WB because it still contains clotting factors and functioning platelets. WB should be used within 4 hours to benefit from optimal platelet function. In patients that require plasma and RBCs, it may be faster to transfuse WB than to organize and thaw individual components (i.e., FFP).

Packed red blood cells

PRBCs are obtained from WB via centrifugation (Fig. 8.7). The cells are stored in CPDA-1 at a temperature between 1°C and 6°C for up to 35 days (Green 2002). If the blood is collected into a bag that contains cell nutrient additive, the shelf life of PRBCs is extended to 42 days.

PRBC transfusions are administered through a blood filter set whose pores are 170 μm in size. Recipients typically require packed cells if they have a condition involving the specific destruction of RBCs. Immune-mediated hemolytic anemia and hemobartonellosis (*Mycoplasma haemofelis*) are two examples of diseases that involve red cell

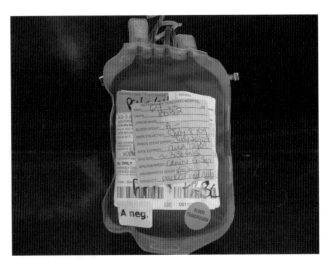

Figure 8.7. One unit of canine PRBCs. The PCV of this unit is 67%.

destruction. Anemia associated with either of these conditions is best treated through transfusion of PRBCs.

PCV may also be used as a guideline for PRBC transfusion. As a general rule, a patient whose PCV is 15% or less and who is showing clinical signs associated with anemia requires a blood transfusion with a PRBC product. Other guidelines for PRBC transfusion are a PCV less than 18% with concurrent red cell destruction and a PCV less than 20% in a dehydrated patient (Mathews 2006a). Recall that dehydrated patients typically present with PCVs that reflect hemoconcentration. If the patient is anemic and dehydrated, it is likely that the patient's true PCV will be less than initial measurements suggest.

Patients with chronic anemia are also candidates for PRBC transfusion. The cardiovascular system in these animals has had time to compensate for their anemia and as such may be overwhelmed by administration of WB. In addition to the cells the animal requires, WB also contributes plasma to the intravascular volume. This may cause volume overload in a compensated animal. It follows that a patient with cardiac insufficiency is a candidate for PRBC transfusion rather than WB.

Platelet products

Blood products are available for use in patients that specifically require platelets. Platelet-rich plasma and platelet concentrate are both commercially available or can be harvested from donated WB via centrifugation. Cost, frequency of use, and shelf life are significant drawbacks associated with platelet products. Platelets must be stored at room temperature because refrigeration interrupts normal platelet function. In addition, the platelets must be kept on a rocker (in continuous motion) and used within 24 hours of collection (Fig. 8.8).

Platelet products are indicated for patients whose platelet numbers or lack of platelet function is so severe that spontaneous bleeding has begun. Petechiae, bleeding gums, epistaxis, or hemorrhage may be appreciated in these patients. Transfusing thrombocytopenic patients with platelet products is possible, but the small number of platelets obtained through the transfusion is typically not enough to be clinically relevant. Where

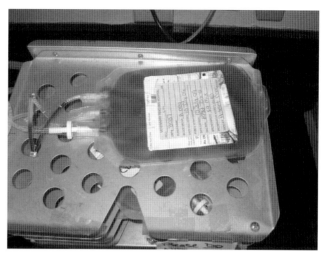

Figure 8.8. One unit of platelet concentrate. This product must be stored in motion and kept on a rocker, gently titrated.

a choice of products is available to the clinician, platelet concentrate is thought to be the more efficient product of the two (Green 2002).

 Nursing considerations

Any transfusion of blood products or blood components can cause adverse reactions in the recipient. The outer surface of RBCs is coated with small structures primarily composed of protein. Most of the animals within a species have the same protein structures at similar locations on their RBCs. Variation in this arrangement does occur within a species, and from this variation arise the different blood types. The structures that are consistent are antigenic. The exceptions in the species have slightly different protein structures at slightly different locations on the surface of their RBCs. The structures present in a smaller proportion of the species are allogenic (Green 2002). Transfusion of one of these blood types to an animal that possesses the other blood type stimulates an immune response in the recipient. The recipient's body produces antibodies in response to the foreign protein. The reaction of the antibody is to bind to the donor antigen. In large numbers, this antigen binding can cause RBCs to clump together. This process is more commonly referred to as agglutination. In severe cases, the immune reaction is severe and immediate; in others, it can be delayed and slightly less severe.

Blood type is an important consideration when any blood component therapy is instituted. Canine patients are split into three categories for the purposes of transfusion medicine. The protein structures found on canine RBCs are referred to as dog erythrocyte antigens (DEAs). DEA 1.1 and DEA 1.2 are antigens found at specific locations on the RBC. Dogs that are lacking antigens at either of those locations are typed DEA 1 negative. Dogs that have antigens at either location are typed DEA 1.1+ or DEA 1.2+. A dog that is positive at either location can receive blood from another dog that is positive at either location. A DEA 1+ dog can also receive DEA negative blood with relative safety. A DEA negative patient *should not* receive DEA positive blood because this can cause a severe immune response from the recipient. If the recipient is receiving DEA positive blood for the first time, it is unlikely that the patient has already formed anti-bodies. For this reason, a noticeable reaction may not arise for several days after the transfusion. If another DEA positive transfusion is given to the patient 7 to 10 days later, the animal has presumably had time to stage an immune response, and it is likely that the reaction to the second transfusion will be severe (Green 2002).

Feline blood types are similar in principle to canine blood types. Cats are either type A, type B, or type AB. Most cats are type A, with type B cats highly represented by the purebred population. Type AB is quite rare. The main difference between canine and feline blood types is that cats do not need an initial transfusion of a foreign blood type to develop antibodies; they are born with the respective antibodies. If a type B cat is transfused with type A blood, it is possible that this single transfusion may cause a severe life-threatening reaction in the recipient (Castellanos et al. 2004).

Immediate transfusion reactions involve destruction of the foreign RBCs. This is an immune-mediated response and involves intravascular destruction of the RBCs. Clinical signs involved with this type of reaction include hemoglobinemia, hemoglobinuria, vomiting, fever, facial swelling, and tachycardia (Mathews 2006a).

Delayed reactions are typically less severe than immediate reactions and may involve pruritus, facial swelling, fever, and seizures. Other adverse reactions are possible even if the recipient's immune system is not stimulated. For example, patients with cardiac insufficiency are susceptible to vascular volume overload with the administration of natural colloids. Clinical signs of volume overload include but are not limited to cough, tachypnea, dyspnea, and vomiting.

Chapter Summary

There are many choices to make when selecting an appropriate fluid for an individual patient. Note that the characteristics associated with the different types of fluid make them appropriate for some situations and inappropriate for others.

Crystalloid solutions are perhaps the most commonly used fluids in veterinary practice. They contain low molecular weight particles and generally have a concentration of sugar or salt. The movement of crystalloid solutions is not restricted, and they flow freely out of the vascular space within a short time of administration. Crystalloids do not contribute to oncotic pressure, but they do contribute to osmotic pressure.

Crystalloid solutions are divided into maintenance fluids and replacement fluids. Replacement fluids are used to treat animals that are dehydrated on presentation and suffering from ongoing losses due to illness. These fluids are isotonic and contain a sodium concentration similar to that of the extracellular space. Some replacement solutions contain buffers and have a pH that has an alkalinizing effect on the patient's blood. Maintenance solutions contain less sodium than replacement fluids and are hypotonic. They are used for maintenance of body water and primarily replenish and maintain the intracellular space.

Colloids are large molecular weight solutions that remain in the intravascular space after administration. They are often used to increase intravascular volume because their oncotic effects draw fluid from other body water compartments.

Synthetic colloids are widely used in small animal practice. When compared with crystalloids, synthetic colloids have an increased cost and greater number of adverse reactions associated with their use. However, if compared with natural colloids, synthetics have a greater shelf life, lower cost, and fewer reactions. Lack of oxygen-carrying capacity and absence of coagulation factors are two drawbacks associated with synthetic colloids.

Natural colloids are beneficial to patients suffering from severe hemorrhage, coagulopathies, and chronic anemia. Although they may elicit adverse reactions in some patients, they have a relatively large margin of safety when used judiciously. Blood products offer the benefits of coagulation factors and oxygen-carrying capacity; a combination not offered by any other type of IV fluid in veterinary medicine.

Canine and feline patients must be typed before administration of blood products. Transfusion of mismatched blood components can elicit severe life-threatening reactions in the recipient.

Small animal practitioners are fortunate to have a wide variety of fluid types from which to build their therapy. Veterinary technicians can provide irreplaceable insight and forethought to the practitioner provided they have a basic understanding of fluid types and their appropriate uses.

Review Questions

1. Identify three important characteristics of crystalloids.
2. Circle the appropriate answer. Maintenance crystalloids contain more/less sodium than replacement crystalloids.
3. The concentration of sodium in hypertonic saline is _____ 0.9% NaCl.
   a. higher than
   b. lower than
   c. the same as
4. Why is hypertonic saline used for fluid resuscitation of hypovolemic patients?
5. Colloids contain large molecular weight particles. Why is this of benefit in fluid therapy?
6. Why must one exercise caution when using HTS or colloids for volume expansion?

Answers to the review questions can be found on page 224 in the Appendix. The review questions are also available for download on a companion website at www.wiley.com/go/donohoenursing.

Further Reading

American Thoracic Society Consensus Statement. 2004. Evidence-based colloid use in the critically Ill. *Am J Resp Crit Care Med* 170:1247–1259.

Bateman, S. 2003. Using synthetic colloids. Proceedings Western Veterinary Conference.

Boldt, J., and H. J. Priebe. 2003. Intravascular volume replacement therapy with synthetic colloids: is there an influence on renal function? *Anesth Analg* 96:376–382.

Brooks, M. B. 2003. Blood component therapy. Clinical use in small animal practice. Proceedings American College of Veterinary Medicine.

Castellanos, I., C. Couto, and T. Gray. 2004. Clinical use of blood products in cats: a retrospective study. *J Vet Intern Med* 18:529–532.

Center, S. 2006. Fluid, electrolyte, and acid-base disturbances in liver disease. In S. DiBartola, ed. *Fluid, Electrolyte, and Acid-Base Disorders in Small Animal Practice*, 437–477. St. Louis: Saunders.

Cohn, L. A., et al. 2007. Response of healthy dogs to infusions of human serum albumin. *Am J Vet Res* 68:657–663.

DiBartola, S., & S. Bateman. 2006. Introduction to fluid therapy. In S. DiBartola, ed. *Fluid, Electrolyte, and Acid-Base Disorders in Small Animal Practice*, 325–344. St. Louis: Saunders

Green, M. 2002. Transfusion medicine. In W. E. Wingfield, ed. *The Veterinary ICU Book*, 189–201. Jackson, WY: Teton NewMedia.

Homma, H., et al. 2005. Small volume resuscitation with hypertonic saline. *J Trauma* 59:266–272.

Logan, J., et al. 2001. Clinical indications for use of fresh frozen plasma in dogs: 74 dogs (October through December 1999). *JAVMA* 218:1449–1455.

Martin, L. 2004. Human albumin solutions in the critical patient. Proceedings International Veterinary Emergency and Critical Care Society.

Mathews, K. 2004. Indications and guidelines for "fluid" management in various situations. Proceedings Western Veterinary Conference.

Mathews, K., and M. Barry. 2005. The use of 25% human serum albumin: outcome and efficacy in raising serum albumin and systemic blood pressure in critically ill dogs and cats. *J Vet Emerg Crit Care* 15:110–118.

Mathews, K. 2006a. Fluid therapy: non-hemorrhage. In *Veterinary Emergency and Critical Care Manual*, 347–372. Guelph, Ontario, Canada: LifeLearn.

Mathews, K. 2006b. Monitoring fluid therapy and complications of fluid therapy. In S. DiBartola, ed. *Fluid, Electrolyte, and Acid-Base Disorders in Small Animal Practice*, 377–391. St. Louis: Saunders

Mathews, K. 2008. The therapeutic use of 25% human serum albumin in critically ill dogs and cats. *Vet Clin North Am Small Anim Pract* 38:595–605.

Mazzaferro, E., E. Rudloff, and R. Kirby. 2002. The role of albumin replacement in critically ill veterinary patients. *J Vet Emerg Crit Care* 12:113–124.

Mensack, S. 2008. Fluid therapy: options and rational administration. *Vet Clin Small Anim* 38:575–586.

Methany, N. 1992. Intravenous therapy. In *Fluid and Electrolyte Balance*, 149–168. Philadelphia: JB Lippincott.

Moore, L. 2003. Crystalloids/Colloids/Oxyglobin/Blood products. Proceedings North American Veterinary Conference.

Rudloff, E., and R. Kirby. 2001. Colloid and crystalloid resuscitation. *Vet Clin North Am* 31:1207–1229.

Sheikh, A., et al. Cerebral effects of resuscitation with hypertonic saline and a new low sodium hype. *Crit Care Med* 24:1226–1232.

Silverstein, D. C. 2009. Daily intravenous fluid therapy. In *Small Animal Critical Care Medicine*, 271–280. St. Louis, MO: Saunders.

Trow, A. et al. 2008. Evaluation of use of human albumin in critically ill dogs: 73 cases (2003-2006). *JAVMA* 233:607–612.

Varicoda, E., et al. 2003 Blood loss after fluid resuscitation with isotonic or hypertonic sodium chloride for the initial treatment of uncontrolled hemorrhage induced by splenic rupture. *J Trauma* 55:112–117.

Wardrop, K. J. 2004. Plasma transfusion in the dog. Proceedings Western Veterinary Conference.

Internet Resources

Product information regarding pentastarch: http://pentaspan.homestead.com/enter.html.

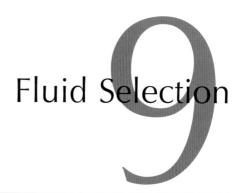

Fluid Selection

Processes Involved in Fluid Selection

This chapter outlines the decision-making process involved in selecting fluid types for specific illnesses. It is true that there is often more than one choice of fluids that is appropriate for any given patient. With this in mind, you should appreciate that the path chosen in each example is but one option in many and used to illustrate the thought process involved.

Fluid selection is an important component of any patient's therapeutic plan. The clinician must consider a number of factors before choosing the fluid type most suitable at the outset of fluid therapy. Recall also that the fluid type used during the initial stages of fluid therapy may not continue to be the ideal fluid type for the patient's dynamic condition and changing needs. For example, a patient that presents in decompensatory shock requires immediate intervention and fluid support. Once this patient has been stabilized, fluid requirements will likely change. In contrast, a patient that presents to the hospital with mild signs of ill health might receive only one type of fluid throughout its stay in the hospital.

Patient Evaluation

Ideally, each patient should benefit from a physical examination before the onset of fluid therapy. Understandably, this examination is not always achievable in the early stages of an emergency. Vascular access often is obtained and fluid therapy instituted *while* the

Fluid Therapy for Veterinary Technicians and Nurses, First Edition. Charlotte Donohoe.
© 2012 Charlotte Donohoe. Published 2012 by John Wiley & Sons, Inc.

clinician is performing a primary evaluation. Nevertheless, the patient's hydration status and perfusion are parameters that need be identified as soon as possible upon presentation.

Perfusion is estimated by evaluation of the animal's mucous membrane (MM) color and capillary refill time (CRT). Heart rate and pulse quality are also indicators of perfusion. Pale MM color, prolonged CRT (>2 seconds), elevated heart rate, and weak pulse pressure are often appreciable in patients whose perfusion is compromised. Body temperature is typically decreased in poorly perfused animals, and the extremities are often cool. These patients require fluid therapy to begin as soon as possible.

Hydration status is estimated through evaluation of MM moisture, skin tent, and ocular position. Animals with tacky or dry MM, prolonged skin tent, and sunken globes are suffering from some degree of dehydration. Mild hydration deficits typically do not require emergency intervention and can be corrected over a longer period of time than poor perfusion. Recall that prolonged dehydration can lead to poor perfusion. In this instance, fluid therapy should begin as soon as possible.

Vomiting and Diarrhea

Vomiting and diarrhea are common ailments for which animals are presented to the veterinary hospital. Body water is lost both through direct expulsions of fluid as well as through lack of intake. The loss of water leads to a decrease in the volume of the extracellular compartment. The fluid lost is isotonic, and there is no shift of water between compartments. The extracellular compartment is the first to be affected, and if the illness is treated before the animal is severely compromised; the other compartments will suffer little to no effects. If water loss is purely the result of the animal being unable to drink, the loss is considered hypertonic because there is no equivalent loss of sodium (Brown and Otto 2008).

Patients whose primary complaints are vomiting and diarrhea tend to show signs of dehydration more slowly than animals that suffer from diarrhea or vomiting secondary to other disease processes. For example, a dog that has recently suffered a dietary indiscretion can tolerate the loss of body water through vomiting far better than a dog whose vomiting is a side effect of septic peritonitis or septicemia.

Clinical signs

Clinical signs associated with vomiting and diarrhea include, but are not limited to, a decrease in body weight, decreased urine output, increased packed cell volume (PCV), and increased total protein (TP). Mild dehydration may not cause an increase in heart rate; however, prolonged dehydration leads to hypovolemia and is reflected by an increased heart rate and weak to thready pulses (Table 9.1). Hypovolemic shock is the stage at which the body's compensatory mechanisms have been overwhelmed by the loss of water and can no longer maintain the blood volume circulating within the vasculature.

Hospitals with advanced monitoring equipment have the capacity to trend the patient's central venous pressure and blood pressure, two parameters that are affected by prolonged dehydration and hypovolemia. Continuous monitoring of these parameters allows for significant insight into fluctuations in patient status. In addition, lactate is a valuable monitoring tool. Hypovolemic animals suffer a decrease in oxygen delivery

Table 9.1 Physical Examination Findings as Related to Degree of Dehydration

Estimated Percentage of Dehydration (%)	Skin Turgor	Mucous Membranes	Heart Rate	Pulse Pressure
<5	No abnormal finding	Moist	Within normal limits	Strong
5	No abnormal finding	Tacky	Within normal limits	Strong
7	Mild to moderate increase in skin tent	Dry	Mild to moderate increase	Strong
10	Moderate to marked increase in skin tent	Dry	Tachycardia	Decreased pulse pressure
12	Marked increase in skin tent	Dry	Tachycardia	Decreased to absent

to their tissues (the result of a decreased circulating volume). The decrease in oxygen delivery forces metabolism to occur in hypoxic conditions. This anaerobic metabolism produces lactate, which can be measured in the animal's blood. Elevated lactate levels are often present in dehydrated patients, but these levels are quick to normalize as fluid therapy progresses.

Gastric fluid is rich in sodium (Na) and chloride (Cl). Vomiting of gastric contents may cause a hyponatremia and hypochloremia. If emesis involves more than just gastric contents, electrolyte imbalances become more complex. Potassium is also lost in vomitus and feces. Decreased or absent food intake is also a cause of potassium loss. Anorexia coupled with the loss of gastrointestinal fluid make hypokalemia a common finding in vomiting and diarrhea patients.

Choosing fluids

Does the patient need fluids?

If an animal is suffering from gastrointestinal upset, it can be mildly or severely affected by the illness. In general, animals whose symptoms have not resolved promptly on their own will need intervention and fluid therapy. It is often the case that patients presented to the emergency hospital with a complaint of persistent vomiting and diarrhea is at a point in their illness where they are in need of fluid therapy. Physical examination will confirm the need for intervention and indicate the urgency with which it must occur. Some patients may present with mild dehydration, whereas others are severely dehydrated, hypovolemic, and experiencing marked electrolyte abnormalities. Regardless of how severely the patient is affected, the fluid therapy plan should begin with the resuscitation and replacement phases and transfer into the maintenance phase as improvements are trended through the patient's vital signs.

What level of intervention is necessary?

Profound dehydration, hypovolemia, and shock are indications for the initiation of the *resuscitation* phase of fluid therapy in vomiting/diarrheic patients. Fluids can be delivered in small volumes (boluses) while the technician diligently reevaluates the animal's vital signs between boluses. Replacement fluids can be delivered in volumes of 10 to 20 mL/kg intravenously (IV) over 15–20 min and repeated as necessary. Technicians must be extra cautious delivering fluid and fluid boluses to patients that are thought to have any degree of cardiac disease. Extra caution is also warranted when delivering fluids to patients with marked hypoalbuminemia.

What goals does the clinician have in mind when prescribing fluid therapy for this patient?

The goal of the resuscitation phase is to restore normal MM color and normal capillary refill time and to improve pulse pressure, heart rate (likely decrease), and mentation. Clinical evaluation of urine output, central venous pressure, blood pressure, and lactate can confirm success of the resuscitation phase of fluid therapy.

Which fluids should be administered?

Several factors must be considered when selecting the type of fluid for a patient. The clinician must decide to what degree the animal is dehydrated and how the animal has lost body fluid. For example, if the animal was involved in an accident and known to have lost a significant amount of blood, the clinician may opt for crystalloid fluids coupled with a blood product. The availability of blood products will obviously dictate the choices made in individual situations. If the animal is found to be hypovolemic and compromised cardiovascularly, the clinician must recall that the patient requires prompt delivery of fluids but also requires fluids that will provide and maintain volume within the intravascular space. In this instance, the clinician might select a crystalloid and deliver it in conjunction with a synthetic or natural colloid.

The fluid selection for a vomiting and diarrhea patient follows the same thought process; consideration must be given to the degree to which the animal is compromised. Blood products are not typically necessary for these patients because there is rarely a significant blood volume lost in the vomiting and diarrheic animal. Crystalloids are an excellent choice because some will remain in the vasculature and most will be distributed to the extravascular space. Furthermore, the vomiting patient is losing body fluid rich in Na^+ and Cl^-. Selecting a fluid that will replenish these electrolytes will benefit the patient.

Replacement crystalloid fluids are isotonic. They are ideal for patients experiencing vomiting and/or diarrhea because they provide water and Na^+. Their Na^+ concentration is very close to that of the extracellular space, the space primarily affected by vomiting and diarrhea. By delivering this type of fluid in the initial stages of therapy, the clinician is able to restore the intravascular volume as well as to correct the animal's dehydration. The constitution of replacement crystalloids also makes them safe for use during resuscitation if needed before the replacement phase of fluid therapy. Maintenance fluids are inappropriate during the initial stages of fluid therapy because they contain an inadequate concentration of sodium.

Consideration must be given to the animal's metabolic status when selecting fluids for resuscitation. Availability of cage-side blood analysis equipment is not widespread, which means that absolute diagnosis of metabolic acidosis or alkalosis is often beyond the clinician's reach. However, many patients that present with vomiting and diarrhea as a primary complaint have some degree of acidosis. As such, they benefit from the use of a buffered solution in their fluid therapy plan.

Plasma-Lyte A, Normosol R, or lactated Ringer solution are all appropriate fluids for the replacement phase of the vomiting/diarrhea patient's fluid therapy plan. These solutions also contain buffers and will help offset acidosis if it is present (Rudloff and Kirby 2001).

In the event of hypovolemia and compromised perfusion, synthetic or natural colloids would be an appropriate choice as an adjunct to the crystalloid fluids. The addition of colloids provides oncotic support and keeps the crystalloids in the vascular space for a longer period of time. Patients that are moderately to severely compromised as a result of their gastrointestinal disturbance may also be suffering from the loss of albumin through their gastrointestinal tract. Colloid boluses should be considered when total proteins drop to less than 4.5 g/dL (Brown and Otto 2008).

Although plasma may be beneficial to the severely compromised patient, whole blood does not impart significant benefits to the vomiting/diarrheic patient. If the patient's gastrointestinal disease includes a perforating ulcer and/or severe anemia, whole blood may be an appropriate product to include in the animal's fluid therapy plan.

By which route should the fluids be delivered?

In mild cases of dehydration, crystalloid fluids can be delivered via any number of different routes. Where possible, fluids may be given by mouth; however, this is not typically possible for patients whose primary complaint is vomiting.

The subcutaneous route is also a suitable means of fluid delivery in mild cases of ill health, but it certainly limits the volume of replacement fluids that can be delivered.

IV delivery of replacement fluids allows the clinician to fine-tune delivery rate and volume and also provides the means to deliver fluid boluses when necessary. In addition, cases that require colloids as part of their therapy may receive them promptly if venous access has already been established for delivery of fluids.

Where IV access is unobtainable, intraosseous catheter placement may be necessary. This route may be useful in stabilizing the patient, facilitating administration of enough fluid to restore intravascular volume and allow the technician to obtain IV access.

The maintenance phase of fluid therapy begins once the animal's hypovolemia has been corrected. Dehydration is corrected more slowly and should be addressed over the following 12 to 24 hours. Ongoing losses such as persistent vomiting and/or diarrhea must be accounted for, and estimated volumes of each should be added to the daily volume of maintenance fluids being delivered.

Maintenance fluids distribute more rapidly than replacement fluids and are used to replenish the extravascular space. IV infusion of maintenance fluids achieves approximately 10% of volume infused as a remainder in the vascular space 1 hour after infusion (Mensack 2008). The solutions commonly used for the maintenance phase of fluid therapy include 0.45% NaCl, 0.45% NaCl with 2.5% dextrose, half-strength lactated Ringer solution with 2.5% dextrose, Normosol M, and Plasma-Lyte 56.

It is not uncommon for critically ill patients to remain on isotonic replacement solutions for the duration of their hospitalization. This is primarily due to the safety of these balanced electrolyte solutions, but it is also a result of the constant fluctuation in fluid balance encountered with critically ill animals.

Continuous monitoring of fluid therapy recipients is mandatory. The technician should be aware of the patient's vital parameters and try to perform at least two temperature, pulse respirations per 24-hour period. Markedly compromised animals require more frequent monitoring.

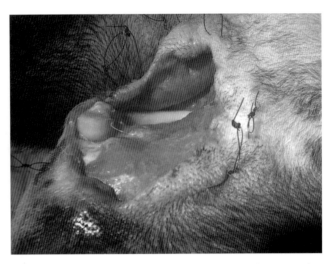

Figure 9.1. This trauma patient sustained multiple severe bite wounds during an altercation with another dog. Boluses of Plasma-Lyte, coupled with a bolus of PENTASPAN, were administered during the resuscitation phase of this patient's fluid therapy. The patient was hypotensive and hypovolemic at presentation.

Trauma

Traumatic injury is a common cause for presentation to an emergency clinic or veterinary hospital (Fig. 9.1). Injuries can be sustained in a wide variety of ways and are not always evident externally during the patient's initial physical examination. Trauma patients most often require fluid therapy as part of their medical intervention, but there is controversy surrounding when these fluids should be delivered and what quantity the patient should receive.

In the event that the animal is able to receive medical attention in the field, the clinician/technician must consider whether or not it is prudent to deliver fluids before arrival at the hospital. The following questions may help guide the medical personnel in their decision regarding initiation of fluid therapy prior to transport to the nearest veterinary facility:

1. **Will initiation of fluid therapy significantly delay the animal's transport to a well-equipped facility?**
   In situations involving a very short trip to a veterinary hospital, the patient may benefit more from prompt arrival than from remaining at the site of the accident to receive fluids. If the trip to the clinic is very short, focusing on arriving at the clinic without delay is likely to be more beneficial to the animal (Sadow 2001).
2. **Will the animal receive a large enough volume of fluids during transport to make it worthwhile delaying transport by setting up fluids?**
   Consider whether or not intervention with fluid therapy will have the time to make a difference during the trip to the clinic. If the animal needs to be transported for quite some distance, it will likely benefit from the fluids feasibly delivered over that time period. A short ride may not even allow enough time for a fluid bolus (10 to 15 minutes). This may lead the clinician to initiate fluid therapy once the animal has arrived at the hospital.

3. **Is the animal experiencing a major hemorrhage?**
   The clinician may elect aggressive fluid therapy in an effort to restore adequate circulation and blood pressure in the early posttrauma period. This is controversial because studies have suggested that aggressive fluid therapy is counterproductive in patients with massive hemorrhage. Raising blood pressure may lead to displacement of a clot that has tenuously formed at the injured site. Studies have suggested that aggressive fluid therapy in the trauma patient can lead to increased hemorrhage and increased mortality (Sadow 2001). To avoid this possibility, it is recommended that fluid therapy be directed toward restoring a low normal blood pressure, effectively supporting circulation but not providing enough pressure to dislodge a beneficial blood clot (Rudloff and Kirby 2008). Recall that the goals of fluid delivery post-trauma should be to minimize blood loss and restore or preserve the water within the body's compartments.
   The emergency database obtained upon arrival at the clinic should always include packed cell volume/total solids (PCV/TS). This simple inexpensive test provides valuable information that can help guide posttraumatic fluid therapy. Trauma patients may have experienced internal hemorrhage that may or may not have ceased by the time the animal arrives at the hospital. PCV/TS provides the clinician with information with regard to blood loss in the following way: A total solids (TS) less than 6.5 g/L in an animal that has recently experienced some form of trauma (but was previously healthy) is suggestive of internal hemorrhage (Rudloff and Kirby 2008). This is true in the presence *or* absence of anemia. The relationship between anemia and hemorrhage is self-explanatory; however; a normal PCV does not rule out hemorrhage as a possibility but may indicate splenic contraction as a result of hemorrhage (Guyton and Hall 2000b). The spleen acts as a reservoir and houses many red blood cells (RBCs) in excess of those used hourly. Blood loss initiates a chain of events including stimulation of the sympathetic nervous system. The sympathetic nervous system causes the spleen and the splenic vessels to contract, thereby forcing the RBCs out of the spleen and into circulation.
   If it is determined that the patient is experiencing a major hemorrhage, whole blood or blood products will be of great benefit to the patient. In the absence of these, the animal will still require fluid therapy to support the cardiovascular system.

4. **Will the animal survive without immediate delivery of resuscitative fluid therapy?**
   A quick examination of the trauma patient provides the clinician with enough information to determine whether or not the injuries are life threatening. In addition, palpation of pulses, evaluation of MMs, and observation of respiratory pattern will communicate the degree to which the animal's cardiovascular system is compromised. The clinician must use this information to determine whether or not the animal's injuries are life threatening and require immediate initiation of fluid therapy as part of the resuscitative efforts before transport.
   Many trauma situations occur in the absence of a mobile veterinary care team, but similar considerations should be made at the veterinary facility that initially sees the patient. Transport of the trauma patient to an emergency or referral hospital should not take place unless the animal is stable. Many tertiary care facilities welcome the referring clinician to call for advice should they require it before transferring a severely traumatised patient.

Fluid choices

Many of the trauma patients that present to a veterinary care facility require some form of fluid therapy. It is important that each patient be considered as an individual and the fluid therapy plan be tailored specifically to that patient. The patient's condition may change rapidly, for better or worse, which dictates that the technician must monitor the animal closely and be prepared to make corresponding changes in fluid delivery rates. It is undesirable to have one standard approach to the treatment of trauma patients whereby all patients receive the same type of fluid at the same rate, regardless of the situation. Judicious use of fluids is even more important because trauma patients are known to be at higher risk of complications that arise from fluid therapy than other patients receiving fluids (Rudloff and Kirby 2008).

Does the animal need fluids?

The need for fluid therapy is determined through the initial physical examination. The examination provides the clinician and technician with an emergency database or baseline vital signs that can help direct fluid delivery. Animals severely compromised by their injuries often have pale or gray MMs, weak pulse pressure, and tachycardia. The presence of these abnormalities suggests hypovolemia and indicates that the animal should receive fluids.

What are the goals of fluid therapy?

Hypovolemia is a common consequence of trauma. Major impact or collision causes damage in a multitude of ways. Physical destruction or disruption of tissue can lead to direct loss of blood and/or maldistribution of blood flow. The goal of fluid therapy, in the initial phases of the emergency, is to replenish the intravascular volume, restore perfusion, and eliminate life-threatening hypovolemia.

Which fluids should be administered?

Crystalloids
Balanced electrolyte solutions are suitable for the resuscitation phase of therapy for the trauma patient. These solutions provide water and electrolytes to the intravascular space and are also distributed to the interstitium over time. Plasma-Lyte 148, Plasma-Lyte A, and Normosol R are examples of fluids commonly used to treat trauma patients.

Caution must be used when delivering these fluids because the patient may have sustained damage to its vasculature. Damage to the vessels allows for leaks and can lead to interstitial edema.

Colloids
Colloids can be used in conjunction with crystalloids to preserve the colloid osmotic pressure within the vasculature. By essentially holding the crystalloids fluids within the intravascular space, colloids can decrease the likelihood of edema formation in the interstitium as well as decrease the amount of crystalloids necessary to replenish the intravascular volume.

Hypertonic saline (HS) is not considered a colloid; however, it may help achieve the goal of intravascular volume replacement in a similar manner. The high salt concentration of HS changes the osmotic force within the vascular space and causes fluid to shift from the interstitium and the intracellular compartment into the intravascular space. This process allows for delivery of a smaller volume of resuscitation fluids and achieves rapid volume replacement in the trauma patient. An added benefit of HS is that it decreases intracranial pressure, which is a helpful side effect if the animal has sustained head trauma (Rudloff and Kirby 2008).

Whole blood

In cases of severe blood loss, it is prudent to transfuse the patient immediately. Unfortunately, it is often the case that the technician does not have the benefit of time and is thus unable to cross-match blood products before delivery. Depending on availability, whole blood or packed red blood cells may be used for transfusion. Hemorrhage is considered life threatening if blood loss falls between 28 and 40 mL/kg in dogs. The same is true of blood loss of 23 to 32 mL/kg in cats (Mathews 2006). Life-threatening hemorrhage can be treated using whole blood. The transfusion can be delivered at a rate of 10 to 22 mL/kg per hour (Day 2006).

Trauma patients are managed differently among clinicians, largely due to the range of products, technical support, monitoring equipment, and expertise available in different clinical settings. By treating each patient as an individual with specific needs and judiciously monitoring and trending their vital signs, the clinician will be better able to select fluids that optimize patient response and expedite recovery.

Pyloric Obstruction

A patient that presents with a pyloric obstruction typically has a predictable electrolyte disturbance in addition to its visible clinical signs. These animals present an interesting opportunity for consideration of fluid selection.

Obstruction at this level of the gastrointestinal tract leads to vomiting and inappetence. Because the obstruction occurs at the pylorus, the vomitus is composed largely of gastric contents. Hydrochloric acid is lost in vomit as well as water, sodium, and potassium. The loss of hydrogen ions contributes to a metabolic alkalosis. In addition, the loss of body water through persistent vomiting leads to dehydration and eventually a decrease in vascular volume.

Many of the illnesses affecting veterinary patients lead to metabolic acidosis. Pyloric obstruction is particularly interesting because it leads to metabolic alkalosis. Rather than the often selected alkalinizing solution, this condition is one that may be treated with an acidifying solution.

Consideration must also be directed toward the particular components lost with gastric vomiting. Hyponatremia and hypokalemia are products of this ailment as well. If one considers that a solution for fluid therapy must initiate correction of the previously mentioned disturbances (metabolic alkalosis, hyponatremia, hypokalemia), then selection of 0.9% NaCl would be a solid choice for patients with pyloric obstruction (Wingfield 2002). Many other gastrointestinal disturbances cause metabolic acidosis and are appropriately treated with a more alkaline solution such as lactate Ringer solution (pH 6.5) or Plasma-Lyte (pH 5.5). In addition to replacing Na losses, 0.9% NaCl is

Table 9.2 Potassium Supplementation Guidelines for Intravenous Fluid Therapy*

Serum Potassium	Total of mEq KCl to Add to 1000-mL Bag
≤2.0	80
2.0–2.5	60
2.5–3.0	40
3.0–3.5	30
3.5–5.5	20

*Potassium should not be administered at rates greater than 0.5 mEq/kg per hour.

more acidic than other popular replacement fluids (pH 5.0). For this reason it is suitable for an animal that is vomiting gastric contents. To address the potassium losses, it is prudent to supplement the 0.9% NaCl with KCl. The rate of KCl replacement depends on the patient's potassium level (Table 9.2).

Chapter Summary

There is more to the decision process than meets the eye with regard to selecting fluids for urgent and emergent cases. Although some clinicians opt for the same fluid type regardless of the condition of the patient, this is not always the best practice. Length of illness, duration of fluid therapy, acid-base status, and cardiovascular status of the patient must be carefully evaluated before initiation of fluid therapy and fluid selection. As with any aspect of fluid therapy, the individual patient must be considered and treated appropriately for its particular set of circumstances.

Review Questions

1. Which patient characteristics can be evaluated to obtain information regarding perfusion status?
2. Evaluation of hydration status or dehydration is somewhat subjective. Which characteristics are measured during this evaluation?
3. A patient presents to the hospital with a complaint of 48 hours of vomiting and diarrhea, as well as a decreased appetite. Is the clinician more likely to prescribe replacement fluids or maintenance fluids?
4. Which fluids might one choose for fluid resuscitation of a vomiting and diarrhea patient?
5. Name three goals of fluid therapy for the trauma patient.

Answers to the review questions can be found on page 224 in the Appendix. The review questions are also available for download on a companion website at www.wiley.com/go/donohoenursing.

Further Reading

Brown, A., & C. Otto. 2008. Fluid therapy in vomiting and diarrhea. *Vet Clin North Am* 38:653–675.

DiBartola, S., & S. Bateman. 2006. Introduction to fluid therapy. In S. DiBartola, ed. *Fluid, Electrolyte, and Acid-Base Disorders in Small Animal Practice*, 325–344. St. Louis: Elsevier.

Guyton, A., & J. Hall. 2000a. Physiology of gastrointestinal disorders. In *Textbook of Medical Physiology*, 10th ed., 764–771. Philadelphia: Saunders.

Guyton, A., & J. Hall. 2000b. Vascular distensibility and functions of the arterial and venous systems. In *Textbook of Medical Physiology*, 10th ed., 152–161. Philadelphia: Saunders.

Mensack, S.2008. Fluid therapy: options and rational administration. *Vet Clin North Am Small Anim Pract* 38:575–577.

Rudloff, E., & R Kirby. 2001. Colloid and crystalloid resuscitation. *Vet Clin North Am* 31:1207–1229.

Sadow, K. 2001. Prehospital intravenous fluid therapy in the pediatric trauma patient. *Clin Pediatr Emerg Med* 2:23–27.

Weinstein, S. 1997. Principles of parenteral fluid administration. In *Plumer's Principles & Practice of Intravenous Therapy*, 6th ed., 317–344. Philadelphia: Lippincott Williams & Wilkins.

Wingfield, W. 2002. *Fluid and Electrolyte Therapy*. In *The ICU Book*, 167–188. Jackson, WY: Teton NewMedia.

Parenteral Nutrition
10

The Decision to Provide Parenteral Nutrition

Veterinary patients in the advanced care setting are faced with many different stressors and a variety of challenges throughout their illness and during their convalescence. The hospital environment itself is far different from what is familiar to a household pet. In addition to the stress of hospitalization, the animal is confronted with illness, limited exercise, and potentially unfamiliar or unpalatable dietary offerings. The multitude of challenges faced by emergency or intensive care patients contributes to changes in their metabolism and changes in their dietary needs. Failing to provide adequate nutrition during these changes sets the stage for malnutrition, impaired healing, and subsequent or additional illness. The fact that a patients' nutritional needs must be addressed despite the adversity of their situation has led to the use of the parenteral route for provision of nutrition in patients that are unable to receive adequate nourishment orally.

Intravenous (IV) nutrition is frequently used in intensive or critical care settings. The two forms in common use are referred to as partial parenteral nutrition (PPN) and total parenteral nutrition (TPN).

Partial Parenteral Nutrition

PPN is an IV fluid mixture that can provide roughly half of a hospitalized animal's caloric requirements (Proulx 2002) (Fig. 10.1). PPN is used in patients perceived to need supplemental nutrition for a period of up to 5 to 7 days (Mathews 2006). It is composed

Fluid Therapy for Veterinary Technicians and Nurses, First Edition. Charlotte Donohoe.
© 2012 Charlotte Donohoe. Published 2012 by John Wiley & Sons, Inc.

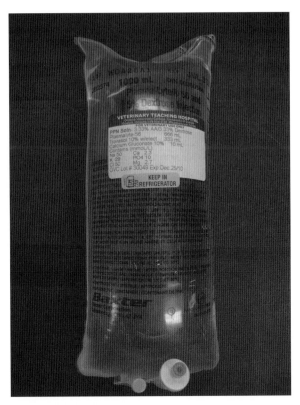

Figure 10.1. Parenteral nutrition solution (PPN) can be compounded by hospital pharmacies. Solutions can be mixed in private practice. Absolute sterile technique is mandatory.

of dextrose, vitamins, amino acids, triglycerides, electrolytes, trace minerals, and lipids. In some cases multivitamins are added to the solution on a per patient basis, and they are injected daily into the fluid bag by the technician. Further adjustments may be made to the mixture according to patient needs. For example, protein content can be increased in animals that require additional protein supplementation. Animals with large draining wounds or animals suffering from hypoalbuminemia may benefit from PPN with higher protein content. In contrast, a patient with hepatic encephalopathy would benefit from slightly lower protein content.

Standard dextrose concentration in PPN solutions is 5% (Freeman and Chan 2006). This component of PPN is also one that can be tailored to individual patients based on their illness and endocrine status. Hyperglycemia is an important concern in critically ill patients, and judicious administration of dextrose, coupled with frequent patient monitoring, is necessary to avoid this complication.

Electrolytes are an important component of PPN, but interestingly they are not delivered as a standard inclusion in all hospitals. Some clinicians prefer to reserve the ability to alter electrolyte administration as the patient's needs change, and as such, they opt to deliver electrolytes as a separate supplement to facilitate adjustment. In general, sodium, potassium, calcium, magnesium, and chloride are provided in the PPN solution. Patients that present in a state of malnutrition may also require supplementation with zinc, chromium, copper, and manganese because these become particularly depleted (Freeman and Chan 2006).

As previously mentioned, vitamins may be added to the PPN as it is mixed or may be administered by the technician on a daily basis. Vitamin supplements should include B vitamins, which are light sensitive. These need to be infused within 6 hours of administration (Mathews 2006). Patients receiving PPN for longer than 4 or 5 days also benefit from vitamins A, D, E, and C.

Total Parenteral Nutrition

TPN is an IV solution designed to provide 100% of a patient's nutritional requirements (Proulx 2002). Its components are similar to that of PPN but with a more substantial protein and calorie content. TPN is formulated with a far higher dextrose concentration than PPN and contains 50% dextrose in the standard solution. TPN is typically reserved for animals that require parenteral nutrition (PN) for longer periods of time, typically longer than 7 days (Proulx 2002). In comparison with PPN, TPN has a greater cost and more complications associated with its use (Freeman and Chan 2006).

Lipids

Lipids are a calorie-dense solution delivered in conjunction with PPN or TPN. They are made up of natural fats, fat-soluble vitamins, triglycerides, phospholipids, and waxes (Crandell 2005). The lipid solution is a concentrated source of energy and essential fatty acids. Its use provides calories that supplement PPN/TPN but does so in a manner that is efficient with respect to the volume delivered (Figs. 10.2 and 10.3).

Administration of lipids to critically ill patients is not undertaken without concern. Side effects such as immunosuppression and hypertriglyceridemia are associated with the use of lipids. Immunosuppression appears to be a more common side effect in critically ill patients that receive lipids as part of their PN (Crandell 2005). These side effects are of particular concern when lipids are made with safflower oil or soybean bases (Freeman and Chan 2006).

Because PPN and TPN can be used in conjunction with, or in the absence of lipids, their use must be well thought out and prescribed by the attending clinician on a case-by-case basis.

Parenteral Nutrition in the Advanced Care Setting

Why is parenteral nutrition necessary?

Weight loss, specifically loss of lean body mass, is detrimental to the health and well-being of any veterinary patient (Fig. 10.4). Animals whose caloric requirements are failing to be met experience delayed wound healing, decreased strength, and even disruption of their immune system. In broader terms, loss of lean body mass has a negative impact on the patient's convalescence, delays their mobility, and lengthens their stay in the hospital.

Critically ill animals expend much of their energy improving their health. Their bodies experience an increased demand for appropriate calories, and as such, their needs are

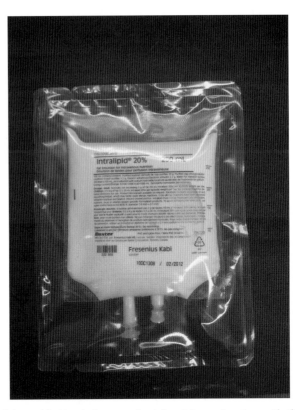

Figure 10.2. A small bag of lipid solution may be infused in conjunction with the parenteral nutrition solution.

different from those of a healthy resting animal. Proulx (2002) differentiates between *simple starvation,* a lack of adequate calories and protein, and *stress starvation,* a lack of adequate calories and protein in conjunction with illness and injury or physiologic stress. Providing a distinction for the starvation that occurs during ill health helps emphasize that a healthy animal has different caloric needs than a sick animal. Loss of body mass and starvation occur more rapidly in the injured or diseased animal than in an otherwise healthy one.

An illness that prevents or discourages an animal from eating for several days sets in motion a chain of events. Inadequate caloric intake causes the body to use its stores of hepatic glycogen. Once these stores have been exhausted, muscles are exploited as a protein source. Specifically, the body mobilizes the muscles' amino acids. The use of muscle mass as a protein source is not without consequence and has been linked with changes in the normal structure of the organs (Proulx 2002). An animal can endure starvation and prolong its survival by using alternative energy sources within its body. However, these means are successful for a finite period of time and not in the face of additional disease. PN can mitigate the effects of the body's catabolic response to starvation by providing an external source of protein and energy. Its use in the critical care setting allows the clinician to decrease the chance that the patient will suffer from disease-related malnutrition throughout its hospitalization. PN may also be used as dietary support for patients that present in an established state of malnutrition.

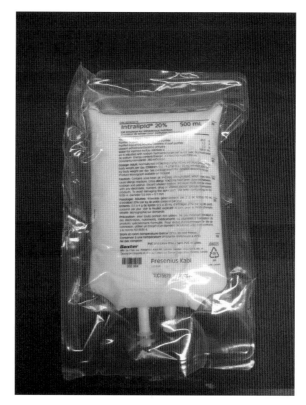

Figure 10.3. Lipids are also available in large bags.

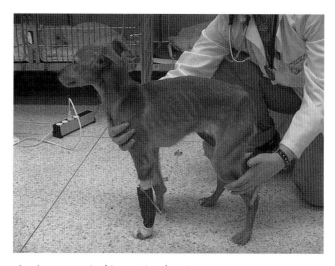

Figure 10.4. Starvation is apparent in this emaciated canine.

When is parenteral nutrition appropriate?

Not every hospitalized patient is a candidate for PN. Many patients are able to maintain their caloric intake through normal eating and drinking. Animals that are inappetent, unable to prehend food, unable to masticate, or have had gastrointestinal disease or procedures involving their gastrointestinal tract may be adequately fed via the enteral route using nasogastric, esophagostomy, gastrotomy, or jejunostomy tubes. Whenever it is possible to feed a patient via the enteral route, one should seize the opportunity to do so. Enteral feeding is known to have a lower incidence of infection and complications than parenteral feeding (McClave et al. 2009). Generally speaking, patients that are candidates for PN are those that cannot tolerate feeding by any of the previously mentioned means.

PN may be the chosen route of nourishment in animals that are currently or are at risk of becoming malnourished, in animals whose history involves 3 days of anorexia, in animals expected to be anorexic for greater than 3 days, or in animals that are at risk of significant loss of muscle mass during their hospital stay.

Timely initiation of PN is an important responsibility carried by the clinician. One must consider that the animal that has been ill for an unknown period of time before admission is likely malnourished and will benefit from prompt administration of PN (Figs. 10.5 and 10.6). In contrast, a patient that has recently sustained trauma was presumably healthy before its accident. Barring any trauma-related damage to the digestive system, PN may be withheld from this patient for a day or two to determine whether it will resume eating on its own.

The physical examination is one approach to evaluating a patient's nutritional status. The combination of the physical examination and the history provided by the patient's owner allows the clinician to develop a reasonable estimation of the presence or absence of malnutrition, starvation, and/or weight loss. Table 10.2 highlights areas that should receive particular attention during the nutritional assessment portion of the physical examination.

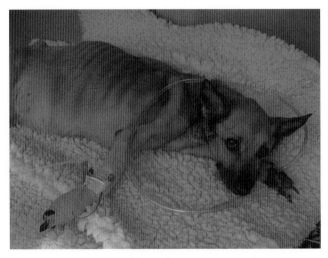

Figure 10.5.   Malnutrition is evident in this dog. This animal has been suffering from its disease for a prolonged period of time. This body condition did not develop suddenly.

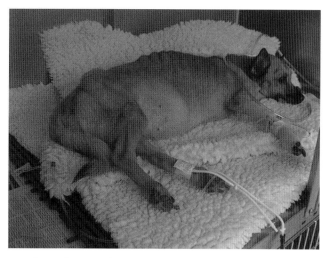

Figure 10.6. Patients suffering from neoplastic disease become cachectic if their disease is left untreated.

Table 10.1 Potential Candidates for Parenteral Nutrition

- >3 d anorexia
- Protracted vomiting
- Gastrointestinal obstruction
- Unprotected airway
- Traumatic injury
- Severe infection
- Sepsis
- Open/Draining wounds
- Acute pancreatitis
- Mechanical ventilation

There is no hard fast rule about when PN should be initiated for a particular patient because each situation is unique (see Table 10.1). What is important to consider is that an animal requiring supplemental nutrition will benefit from the administration of that nutrition as early as possible. In some cases, this must be by the parenteral route. Studies have shown that despite the complications often associated with PN, it is preferable to begin feeding parenterally than to delay feeding until the enteral route is available (Powell-Tuck 2007).

Parenteral nutrition administration

PN must be administered in specific ways. The method chosen by a particular veterinary health care team is decided based on the materials available to them. Labor is also

Table 10.2 Physical Examination Features Suggestive of Malnutrition

Weight	As per owner/medical records
	Weight loss
Muscles	Muscle wasting
	Overt signs of weakness
Hair coat	Dull
	Poor quality
	Lack of grooming
Wounds	Presence of old wounds
	Delayed wound healing
Eyes	Sunken eye position
Organs	May be decreased in size

an important variable that affects the safe administration of PN. Most advanced care settings are well equipped, both with adequate numbers of trained staff and with appropriate materials, to deliver IV feeding safely to their patients. Smaller hospitals, in particular those that do not offer 24-hour care, may have a more difficult time making arrangements that are safe for the patient. PN is a very useful tool in veterinary medicine, but it must not be undertaken without appropriate patient supervision. Delivery of PN with IV fluids over a period of time when the clinic is not staffed with a technician (overnight) leaves the patient vulnerable to a host of complications.

Catheter selection

PN can be administered through an IV catheter. Because the catheter will most likely be in place for several days, it is important to choose a material that has a lower tendency to cause IV damage. Thrombus formation is a concern during PN administration due not only to the presence of the IV catheter but also to the high osmolarity of the solution being infused. The osmolarity of the infusate can cause irritation and inflammation within the cannulated vessel. The catheter causes a direct physical irritation to the lumen of the vessel within which it is seated. The physical damage predisposes the vessel to develop a thrombus.

Some materials have been found to be less irritating to the intravascular lining and thus less thrombogenic than others. Many studies have been undertaken to determine materials suitable for use in long-term indwelling IV catheters. The overall consensus is that silicone and polyurethane catheters have a low incidence of associated thrombus formation and intravascular irritation. These catheter materials are recommended for use with PN infusions (Proulx 2002). Teflon is an example of a catheter material that is thrombogenic (Tan 2003). Polyethylene and polyvinyl chloride catheters are also not recommended for use with PN infusions (Freeman and Chan 2006).

A human study involving 190 oncology patients investigated the complication rate associated with polyurethane catheters. A total of 206 catheters were placed, and the average patient stay was 101 days. The results demonstrated that the complication rate was low; 1 catheter was considered infected of 12 that were removed, and only one thrombosis was recorded (Volkow et al. 2003). Another study involved the IV placement of implants in the femoral veins of rats. The researchers compared silicone, GORE-TEX, and stainless steel implants with respect to vascular irritation and thrombus formation. The implants were left in place for 4 weeks, at which point the vessels were evaluated. The silicone implants had a rare incidence of thrombi and elicited mild perivascular inflammation. The GORE-TEX and stainless steel implants caused moderate amounts of thrombi and moderate perivascular inflammation (Melvin et al 2010). By selecting catheters known to be made with nonthrombogenic material, the technician can decrease the likelihood of catheter-related complications while administering PN.

Catheter sites and solution sets

Catheter sites must be selected with consideration of the PN being delivered. It is necessary to deliver TPN via central venous catheter, but PPN may be delivered through a peripheral catheter.

TPN is a calorie-dense fluid that is hypertonic to blood. Its delivery into a peripheral vein leaves the patient at a higher risk for thrombophlebitis and vascular irritation. A central line provides a safer route for delivery of TPN and is commonly placed in a jugular or saphenous vein. Despite the peripheral location of the saphenous vein, a long catheter fulfills the requirement of a central line when its tip lies in the proximal vena cava. The delivery of TPN into such a large vessel decreases the risk of vascular irritation. Whenever possible, the jugular vein should be selected over the saphenous site because hind limb catheters are contaminated more easily due to their proximity to patient waste (urine/feces).

Multilumen central lines offer the added advantage of separate lumens to dedicate to individual fluids. One lumen can be labeled TPN and used exclusively for its delivery. This exclusivity maintains an infusion line with a decreased number of opportunities for bacterial contamination: The absence of line invasions, medication administrations, and blood draws preserves the integrity of the ports and IV line.

PPN is a more versatile product in the sense that it may be delivered via central venous catheter *or* peripheral catheter. A small-gauge catheter (preferable to larger gauge) in the cephalic or saphenous vein can accommodate PPN delivery. A drawback to using a short peripheral catheter is that the line can rarely be dedicated for the explicit use of PN. The technician should strive to provide a catheter that can be labeled solely for nutrition so that additional invasions of the line are limited, if not entirely eliminated. (Ambulatory canine patients require lines to be invaded for saline flushes when being removed from their cages for walks.) In the event that the peripheral catheter is the sole IV access in the patient, a three-pronged port may be used to allow multiple lines to feed into one catheter. In essence, the PN line is still dedicated, and the contact with other IV fluids is kept to a minimum because the three-pronged port is attached directly to the catheter. The infusions mix for a brief period as they pass through the catheter into the vein. A special technique is observed during medication administration in this instance. The PN line and the additional port/line are clamped and flushed with heparinized saline, and the medication is administered and followed by an additional flush.

A 1.2-µm inline filter can be included in the infusion set to avoid any clumps of lipid or large particles from the PN solution being administered to the patient. PN lines should be changed frequently to diminish the possibility of contamination. Each hospital should develop its own protocol with respect to management of PN lines. As a guideline, it is recommended that TPN/PPN lines be changed every 24 to 48 hours (Matthews 2006; Proulx 2002). As an adjunct to this strategy, the technician can make an effort to hang 24 hours worth of PN at a time. In so doing, the entire solution system can be replaced in a timely manner. Patients that are not having their solutions sets changed every day should at least have the catheter bandages removed and the catheter site inspected daily. PN lines and ports can be wiped using a gauze square soaked in an antibacterial solution to maintain cleanliness between line changes. Should lines become contaminated with any organic material, they should immediately be replaced.

Volumes and administration

The goal of nutrition therapy is to eradicate malnutrition if evident at time of presentation, to provide calories and energy to avoid malnutrition as a result of illness, and to prevent loss of lean body weight during hospitalization. To determine how much an animal requires during its illness, formulas have been created to facilitate calculation of a patient's PN needs. There is variation with respect to clinician preference, and not all hospitals use an identical formula. However, the notion of energy requirements at rest and energy requirements during the stress of illness is widely accepted and involved in the determination of a patient's PN needs.

Before determining the animal's food requirement during illness, it is necessary to have an idea of the animal's caloric requirement in good health. The following formula is used to determine the resting energy requirement (RER) of an individual animal:

$$RER = 70 \times (\text{weight in kg})^{0.75} \text{ (Freeman and Chan 2006)}$$

In the event that calculation of an exponent is not available, the formula can be changed to a slightly simpler format that provides a reasonable alternative:

$$RER = (30 \times \text{weight in kg}) + 70 \text{ (Mathews 2006)}$$

The simplified version is used for patients weighing between 2 and 25 kg.

Thoughts surrounding caloric requirements during illness are varied. Some suggest that the RER must be multiplied by a predetermined factor that corresponds to the degree of illness experienced by the patient. Others argue that a predetermined number is not suitable for all patients and that it is equally beneficial to start the infusion at a rate that satisfies the RER and make changes to the PN rate based on patient response. At this time, both approaches are practiced and appear to be used based on clinician preference.

Upon initiating nutrition therapy, the technician is also responsible for carrying out orders corresponding to administration rates. The infusions are delivered in conjunction with crystalloid fluids in most patients. The technician must monitor fluid administration with due diligence because infusion pumps can be confused and infusion rates can be inadvertently reset in busy hospitals. Each infusion rate should be checked hourly. The technician should also be aware of the total volume of fluids received by the patient on an hourly as well as a daily basis.

Due to the calorie-dense content of TPN, this infusion should be slowly introduced to the patient. Gradual introduction allows the animal's metabolism to become accustomed to the altered content of nutrients in the blood. TPN infusions should also be weaned gradually and should not be suddenly discontinued (Proulx 2002).

Complications

Medication administration and fluid therapy are never undertaken without the knowledge that complications can arise. Proper education surrounding possible complications is an important step in preventing their occurrence. It is most important that the technician administering care to the critically ill patient be familiar with the types of complications that are most likely to occur with each type of therapy. Knowing which problems are commonly associated with PN allows the technician to perform efficiently and to troubleshoot small changes in patients' vitals and general well-being.

Complications associated with PN generally fall into one of two categories: mechanical or physiologic. Mechanical complications are often a specialty of the advanced care technician because she or he operates many different forms of equipment, catheters, and devices every day. Physiologic complications can be of greater consequence to the patient because they reflect changes that have already begun to affect the animal's health. The threat of these complications is the reason for the diligent patient monitoring carried out by the advanced care technician. She or he must be able to alert the clinician to slight changes in the patient to permit prompt tailoring of the nutritional therapy prescription.

Mechanical complications

Mechanical complications encountered during nutritional therapy are similar to those involved with any IV infusion. Most often, they are related to a structural compromise of the infusion catheter. Peripheral catheters are subjected to varying degrees of patient movement and can be dislodged, kinked, disconnected from the fluid line, or even accidentally removed from (or by) the patient. To decrease the likelihood of any of these difficulties, the catheter must be placed with much attention to positioning and to securing the catheter to the patient. Any compromise of sterility behooves the technician to remove the catheter and choose a new site. Disconnection of the PN line from the catheter may allow the catheter to be salvaged, but this must be determined on a case-by-case basis depending on the degree to which the catheter has been exposed. If sterility is compromised, the catheter should be removed. Any event involving disconnection of lines from the catheter requires that new infusion lines replace those previously attached to the bag in use.

Central lines fall prey to similar mechanical difficulties as peripheral lines. Jugular catheters also have the potential to kink, become obstructed, or disconnected from infusion lines. It is less likely for central lines to be inadvertently removed; however, it *is* possible. Because placement of central lines is a technically demanding and time-consuming practice, it is important that any opportunity to avoid replacement of these catheters be seized. Although we strive to maintain central lines in place, it is of significant importance that any problematic lines be removed as soon as they are identified as a possible source of infection.

Infection

IV catheters can be a source of infection in any patient. The integument is host to a number of microbes that are for the most part harmless to the healthy individual. However, failure to properly cleanse the skin before catheter insertion in an immune compromised or ill animal allows for inoculation of bacteria during catheter placement.

Diligent use of sterile technique during placement contributes to catheter safety by significantly reducing the probability of contamination. Maintenance of clean catheter bandages and an unsoiled catheter site also contributes to catheter health in the sense that bacterial populations are kept to a minimum and are less likely to invade the puncture site.

Failure to adhere to strict aseptic technique is not exclusively responsible for catheter-related infections. Presence of a foreign material, such as an indwelling catheter, within the vessel initiates a response by the patient's body. This is particularly prominent in long-term catheters. A coating develops around the catheter a short while after it has been seated within the vessel. It is thought that the body attempts to sequester the foreign material within its vessel (Lloyd 1997). The film that coats the catheter is primarily made of fibrin. It is also able to form a fibrous extension at the catheter tip. Opinions vary with respect to the degree to which the fibrin sheath is responsible for catheter-related infection. A study by the American Pediatric Surgical Association in 1991 concluded that the fibrous film surrounding the catheter protected the catheter by keeping the number of adherent bacterial populations in check (Lloyd 1997). Current thought suggests the presence of fibrin sheath provides an ideal spot to which micro thrombi and opportunistic bacteria can adhere. The combination of a foreign object and a hypertonic infusate present within a vessel sets the stage for lumen irritation and thrombus formation. Thrombi that adhere to the fibrous coating surrounding the catheter provide an ideal site for future infection (Opilla 2008).

PN infusions are thought to put patients at risk for bloodstream infections. It is difficult to pinpoint which facet of nutrition therapy is most responsible for this tendency. Infection can be a result of poor sterile technique during catheter placement, microbial contamination during preparation of the infusate, contamination of the PN solution at time/point of use, catheter contamination, or patient susceptibility due to immunosuppression or other metabolic complications.

Hyperglycemia

Regardless of the circumstances surrounding the use of PN, there is an associated risk for development of hyperglycemia. It is thought that hyperglycemia is the most common metabolic complication associated with the use of PN in veterinary patients (Freeman and Chan 2006). Hyperglycemia is a disturbance with consequences that affect many body systems. Its negative effects on the heart are caused by vasoconstriction and inflammation. In addition, hyperglycemia causes alterations in quantities of free fatty acids. These acids are damaging to the cells of the myocardium (King et al. 2007).

Hyperglycemia and brain injury have an intricately woven relationship. Opinions differ with respect to whether hyperglycemia worsens the brain injury or whether its presence is a sign of the presence of significant injury. Despite these opposing theories, there is agreement that hyperglycemia in brain-injured patients is linked to a poor prognosis (King et al. 2007).

Elevated blood glucose in critically ill patients causes further complications by stimulating the coagulation cascade and altering the inflammatory mechanism. The disruption of normal inflammatory processes has multiple consequences, not the least of which is an increased risk of infection. Hyperglycemia alters the inflammatory process and reduces its ability to respond appropriately to bacterial contamination. The result is that bacteria populations are able to grow with little disruption. In this way, hyperglycemia reduces an animal's ability to fight infection.

Two main mechanisms are responsible for the development of hyperglycemia during nutrition therapy. The first involves the composition of the PN solution. There is a direct link between the concentration of dextrose in the PN infusion and the patient's blood glucose level. PN solutions containing higher concentrations of dextrose lead to elevations in patient blood glucose.

The second set of circumstances that leads to hyperglycemia involves the animal's response to stress and the physiologic changes associated with this response. One of the body's responses to stress or severe illness is to release surplus cortisol and catecholamines. One of the important functions of these hormones is to cause an increase in blood glucose levels.

Understandably, a critically ill patient whose body is responding to the stress of their illness and whose primary source of nutrition contains a significant amount of dextrose is a high-risk candidate for hyperglycemia. The body's response to stress is a factor that is beyond the control of the animal's caregivers. Instead, the clinical team must focus on the delivery of PN, tailoring its ingredients to suit patient needs. Avoidance of dextrose overfeeding is key to minimizing the occurrence of hyperglycemia. Provision of dextrose at a rate of 4 mg/kg per minute or less is recommended (Btaiche and Khalid 2004).

Hypoglycemia

Hypoglycemia is an avoidable complication associated with PN. It is typically encountered during discontinuation of PN rather than throughout therapy. Abrupt cessation of the PN infusion leaves insufficient time for the body to adapt to the decrease in dextrose previously received IV. Patients diagnosed with liver disease, malnutrition, or hypothyroidism are at an increased risk of developing hypoglycemia during withdrawal of PN (Btaiche and Khalid 2004).

Hypoglycemia associated with discontinuation of PN occurs soon after the infusion has been stopped. Glucose monitoring is important, particularly within the first hour that the patient is off PN. Drops in blood glucose can be avoided by gradually weaning the animal off the infusion rather than abruptly stopping it. Slowly decreasing the fluid rate over 1 to 2 hours should be sufficient to avoid hypoglycemia in most patients.

Refeeding syndrome

Refeeding syndrome is an uncommon complication associated with PN. The fact that it can be life threatening makes it an important inclusion in the PN discussion despite its infrequency.

Several metabolic disturbances can arise at the outset of PN therapy. Providing nutrition to a body that has been without for an extended period of time causes a spike in insulin production and release. Insulin causes potassium and glucose to move from the extracellular space into the intracellular space. It also causes magnesium and phosphates to move in the same direction. As a result, the extracellular space develops a deficit of these important electrolytes. Hypophosphatemia, hypokalemia, and hypomagnesemia are the primary disturbances involved in refeeding syndrome.

Clinical signs of hypophosphatemia include weakness and intestinal ileus. In severe cases red cell hemolysis and thrombocytopenia have also been documented as clinical signs of hypophosphatemia.

Patients that develop hypokalemia may develop signs such as muscle weakness, polyuria, and polydipsia. Ventroflexion of head and neck may be witnessed in some cats.

Cardiac function is also affected by severe hypokalemia and can manifest as supraventricular or ventricular arrhythmias (DiBartola and Autron de Morais 2006).

The effects of hypomagnesemia are widespread and difficult to specify. However, two important considerations for the technician are the role of magnesium in cardiac contractility and in nerve transmission. Depletion of extracellular magnesium can lead to cardiac arrhythmias and muscle spasms. Muscle spasms due to hypomagnesemia are uncommon in canine and feline patients.

Vitamin imbalances are also a component of refeeding syndrome. The spike in insulin observed on initiation of PN also results in increased synthesis of proteins. Thiamine is needed for this synthesis, and the overwhelming demand that occurs with refeeding syndrome can lead to a thiamine deficiency (Abood et al. 2006).

Refeeding syndrome can be avoided in most veterinary patients by beginning the PN infusion slowly and gradually increasing the patient's caloric intake. Additional strategies for circumventing this complication are to administer multivitamins in conjunction with the TPN or PPN and to monitor electrolytes regularly throughout nutrition therapy. In so doing, electrolyte disturbances can be identified early on and promptly treated.

Chapter Summary

PN is a useful tool in the advanced and critical care setting. Many veterinary patients lack the desire to eat during a bout of severe illness. Other patients have the desire to eat but not the physical ability. PN provides a route for these patients to receive calories and vitamins despite their medical conditions.

PN can be formulated to provide a percentage of the patient's daily caloric requirements or the entire caloric requirement. Lipids and vitamins are a beneficial addition to the base formulas of PPN and TPN.

As with any form of IV therapy, complications can arise due to the provision of nutrition through an IV catheter. Diligence with cleanliness and sterile technique are mandatory when working with PN bags, fluid lines, and catheters.

Review Questions

1. What is parenteral nutrition?
2. What is the difference between TPN and PPN?
3. When should PN be considered for a particular patient?
4. Identify four complications potentially associated with delivery of PN.
5. What is the refeeding syndrome?

Answers to the review questions can be found on pages 224–225 in the Appendix. The review questions are also available for download on a companion website at www.wiley.com/go/donohoenursing.

Further Reading

Abood, S., M. McLoughlin, et al. 2006. Enteral nutrition. In S. DiBartola, ed. *Fluid, Electrolyte, and Acid-Base Disorders in Small Animal Practice*, 601–619. St. Louis: Saunders.

Btaiche, I., & N. Khalid. 2004. Metabolic complications of parenteral nutrition in adults. Part 1. *Am J Health Syst Pharm* 61:1938–1949.

Chittick, P., & R. J. Sherertz. 2010. Recognition and prevention of nosocomial vascular device and related bloodstream infections in the intensive care unit. *Crit Care Med* 38(8 Suppl):S363–372.

Crabb, S., & L. Freeman, et al. 2006. Retrospective evaluation of total parenteral nutrition in cats: 40 cases (1991–2003). *J Vet Emerg and Crit Care* 16:S21–S26.

Crandell, D. 2005. Use of lipids in parenteral nutrition. Proceedings IVECCS; Atlanta, GA; 527–529.

DiBartola, S., & H. Autron de Morais. 2006. Disorders of potassium: hypokalemia and hyperkalemia. In S. DiBartola, ed. *Fluid, Electrolyte, and Acid-Base Disorders in Small Animal Practice*, 91–121. St. Louis: Saunders.

Freeman, L., & D. Chan. 2006. Total parenteral nutrition. In S. DiBartola, ed. *Fluid, Electrolyte, and Acid-Base Disorders in Small Animal Practice*, 584–600. St. Louis: Saunders.

King, G., M. Knieriem, et al. 2007. Hyperglycemia in critically ill patients. *Compend Contin Educ Pract Vet* 29:360–362.

Lloyd, D. 1997. Central venous catheters for parenteral nutrition: a double-edged sword. *J Pediatr Surg* 32:943–948.

Mathews, K. 2006. Nutritional support for the injured or diseased cat and dog. In *Veterinary Emergency and Critical Care Manual*, 499–519. Guelph, Ontario, Canada: LifeLearn.

McClave, S., R. Martindale, et al. 2009. Guidelines for the provision and assessment of nutrition support therapy in the adult critically ill patient. *J Parenter Enteral Nutr* 33:277–316.

Melvin, M., et al. 2010. Silicon induces minimal thromboinflammatory response during 28-day intravascular implant testing. *ASAIO J.* 56:344–348.

Opilla, M. 2008. Epidemiology of bloodstream infection associated with parenteral nutrition. *Am J Infect Control* 36:S173 e5–8.

Parker, J. W., and R. W. Gaines Jr. 1995. Long-term intravenous therapy with use of peripherally inserted silicone-elastomer catheters in orthopaedic patients. *J Bone Joint Surg Am* 77:572–577.

Pasquel, F., et al. 2010. Hyperglycemia during total parenteral nutrition. *Diabetes Care* 33:739–740.

Powell-Tuck, J. 2007. Nutritional interventions in critical illness. *Proceedings of Nutrition Society* 66:16–24.

Proulx, J. 2002. Nutrition in critically ill animals. In W. E. Wingfield, ed. *The Veterinary ICU Book*, 202–217. Jackson, WY: Teton NewMedia.

Stratman, R., C. Martin, et al. 2010. Candidemia incidence in recipients of parenteral nutrition. *Nutr Clin Pract* 25:282–289.

Tan, R., A. Dart, et al. 2003. Catheters: a review of the selection, utilisation and complications of catheters for peripheral venous access. *Aust Vet J* 81:136–139.

Volkow, P., et al. 2003. Polyurethane II catheter as long-indwelling intravenous catheter in patients with cancer. *Am J Infect Control* 31:392–396.

11

Blood Transfusions and Blood Component Therapy

Transfusion medicine is a standard of care in emergency and specialty practices. As the knowledge base in the field has grown, transfusions have been made safer through the development of fast, accurate, user-friendly point-of-care blood typing equipment and cross-matching procedures. Although transfusion of blood and blood products is never without associated risks, pretransfusion testing, donor screening, and proper sample handling contribute to the safe use of blood component therapy in all types of veterinary care settings.

Blood Components

Whole blood (WB) is the term used to describe blood that has been collected from a donor and has remained intact with respect to the cells and plasma it contains. It is mixed with an anticoagulant and preservative to maintain its integrity but otherwise has been unchanged.

Blood components are the products derived from WB that have been separated, typically by centrifugation, and preserved in smaller volumes. The goal of centrifuging WB is to end up with a specific cell population or fluid type in the highest concentration or purest form possible. For example, WB is often separated into a unit of packed red blood cells (PRBC) and a unit of fresh plasma (FP). Different descriptors are used for the plasma component as its composition and function change according to how and when it is processed. Platelet-rich plasma (PRP), platelet concentrate (PC), and cryoprecipitate (Cryo) are also blood components yielded by the centrifugation of WB.

Fluid Therapy for Veterinary Technicians and Nurses, First Edition. Charlotte Donohoe.
© 2012 Charlotte Donohoe. Published 2012 by John Wiley & Sons, Inc.

Feline blood donation yields smaller volumes of WB than canine donations due to the smaller size of the donor. WB is still divided into components, but the process is usually limited to production of a unit of PRBCs and a unit of plasma.

Blood transfusion or blood component therapy can involve the administration of one or more of the previously mentioned components to an individual patient. In contrast, the use of blood components also allows one donation to potentially benefit more than one patient by using the separated components to treat different conditions in separate animals.

Blood and blood products are obtained from a source that is suitable for the needs of an individual practice. Blood banks are organizations that provide blood products to veterinary practices throughout North America. Most are accessible online, which facilitates cost comparison and simplifies the ordering process.

Alternatives to blood banks are available. Individual veterinary practices must decide what is appropriate for their situation. Consideration should be given to the availability of suitable storage options for blood products, client base, frequency of emergency admissions, and presence or absence of equipment needed for the safe administration of blood products. In smaller, quieter practices, it may be feasible to have a list of available donor animals that can be on call for the occasional emergency requiring blood. Alternatively, a practice may benefit from hosting its own blood donor program, either using resident animals or animals whose owners volunteer them to participate in the program.

Blood Donors

To preserve the health and well-being of canine and feline donors, it is imperative that these animals be screened before selection for donation. Guidelines have been developed to assist in donor selection.

Canine blood donors

Because blood collection is usually a quick and simple process, dogs with an easygoing personality often do not need the aid of chemical restraint for their donation. Canine donors should be outgoing dogs, comfortable with restraint, and have no history of aggression. Dogs that meet other donor criteria but have minor anxiety can still enter the blood donor program because mild sedation is often all that is necessary to overcome their apprehension.

Canine donors should be between 1 and 7 years of age and weigh at least 22 kg (50 lbs). In addition to the personality and age requirements, certain health criteria must also be met. Potential donors should have no history of heart disease or seizures. Physical examination should not document any abnormal findings that may be related to potential or progressive disease conditions (i.e., enlarged lymph nodes, bumps that may be undefined tumors). Preventive medications are acceptable for potential donors, but other than heartworm and other antiparasitic medication, donors should not be taking medication regularly.

Feline blood donors

Unlike their canine counterparts, selection of potential feline donors is not as personality dependent. Cats that are notoriously extremely fractious are certainly not ideal candidates for blood donors. However, it is rare to find a feline donor that is not objectionable on some level. For this reason, feline blood collection is always undertaken with the benefit of chemical restraint. Standard operating procedures may vary from one donor program to the next. Feline donors may receive injectable sedation or anaesthetic or receive full general anaesthesia with inhalants.

Feline donors should have a body weight that is not less than 4.5 kg (10 lbs). The cat should be between 1 and 7 years of age. Other criteria are much the same as those for canine donors. The potential donor should have no history of heart disease or murmur and no history of seizure activity. Preventive medication is acceptable, but the cat should not be receiving other medication regularly.

Prescreening potential donors

Once the initial donor selection criteria have been met, the candidates should undergo routine blood work, and vaccines status should be examined and updated if necessary. Blood work should consist of a complete blood count, a platelet count, and a full biochemical profile.

Canine donors should be screened for von Willebrand factor disturbances, tickborne disease (i.e., babesiosis, Lyme disease), heartworm disease, and brucellosis. In addition, it is prudent to consider diseases that may be endemic to a particular geographic location and screen for these if possible. Donors should be vaccinated for distemper, rabies, and parvovirus as a minimum standard of care. Fecal testing and thorough physical examination should confirm the absence of parasitic infestations.

Potential feline donors should be screened for common viral infections such as feline leukemia virus and feline immunodeficiency virus. *Mycoplasma haemofelis* and heartworm screening are also recommended for potential feline blood donors. Cats should be fully vaccinated against rabies, feline viral rhinotracheitis, calicivirus, and panleukopenia. Fecal testing and physical examination should be performed to ensure the candidate is parasite free. All donors should be blood typed before admission to a blood donor program.

Blood Types

Different blood types exist within the canine and feline species, respectively. It is important to identify the blood type of each recipient and each donor. Transfusion of a blood component that differs from that of the recipient can lead to severe and sometimes fatal transfusion reactions in the recipient.

Canine blood types

Red blood cells (RBCs) are coated with antigens, structures made of protein and complex carbohydrates. An antigen is a material that causes antibody production when introduced into the body. Canine blood types are classified in a system that identifies specific dog erythrocyte antigens (DEAs). There are seven different blood groups categorized by this system. Each blood type is grouped according to the location of the antigen on the RBC membrane. The positions on the membranes are organized using a numeric system. Dogs may or may not have antigens at the locations identified as 1.1, 1.2, 3, 4, 5, and 7, and they can also be positive or negative for the *Dal* antigen (Tocci and Ewing 2009). DEA 1.1 and DEA 1.2 are the most clinically relevant antigens with respect to transfusion medicine. DEA 1.1 negative dogs are those that do not have an antigen at the location 1.1. Dogs that are DEA 1.1 positive have an antigen at that location. DEA 1.1 negative dogs that receive a transfusion from a DEA 1.1 positive donor will start producing anti-DEA 1.1 antibodies shortly after receiving the transfusion. The antibodies adhere to the foreign RBCs and eventually destroy them. This type of reaction is known as a delayed reaction and typically not life threatening. More severe transfusion reactions involve much more acute destruction of RBCs; they are immediate and life threatening.

The nomenclature associated with blood types is most commonly abbreviated to A– or A+ based on the DEA 1.1 and 1.2 locations. An A– patient does not have an antigen at either location, but an A+ patient can have an antigen at either or both locations. For this reason, clarification of donor/recipient compatibility based on blood typing performed using typing cards should be carried out by way of cross matching. A+ dogs can safely receive A– blood because there is no foreign antigen to which they react. The opposite situation, an A– dog receiving A+ blood, introduces RBCs with antigens at locations that are foreign to the A– dog, and an immune reaction is initiated. Because dogs are not born with an anti DEA 1.1 antibody, an A– dog can usually safely receive one A+ transfusion but no further A+ transfusions subsequent to that (Tocci and Ewing 2009). Dogs with the A– blood type are considered universal donors because they can safely donate to A– or A+ recipients.

Feline blood types

The feline blood type classification system identifies cats as having blood type A, B, or AB. The most frequently occurring blood type in domestic feline patients in the United States is type A (Green 2002). In contrast to canine counterparts, some cats are *born* with preformed antibodies that will attack foreign blood types. Cats that have type B blood possess anti-A antibodies and can mount a life-threatening reaction to their first transfusion of type A blood (recall that A– dogs can potentially receive one transfusion of A+ blood due to the absence of preformed antibodies).

Type A cats are sometimes but not always born with anti B antibodies. Roughly 30% of type A cats have these antibodies before ever receiving a transfusion of type B blood (Green 2002). Whereas B cats transfused with incompatible blood products generally have severe reactions, A cats more often experience a milder reaction.

As the science of transfusion medicine progresses, more antigens are being discovered. So far, these have been unrelated to the DEA and A and B antigens in dogs and cats, respectively. For example, the DAL antigen in dogs was first reported as recently as 2002 (Blais 2002) and published in 2007. At the moment, DAL antigen negative dogs are rare. Because DAL antigen typing is not yet widely practiced, it is possible that many DAL-negative patients may receive an initial transfusion of DAL-positive blood. As such, they will become sensitized to the DAL antigen and risk severe hemolytic transfusion reactions in the future.

Similarly, the discovery of the Mik antigen in cats was first presented in 2005 (Weinstein 2007). The anti-Mik antibodies are also thought to be naturally occurring in cats, similar to the anti-A antibodies in type B cats.

Blood Typing

Due to the potential for life-threatening transfusion-associated reactions in recipients, blood typing before transfusion is a necessity. Undoubtedly, situations arise that dictate immediate delivery of blood products and do not allow the clinical team the luxury of time for compatibility testing. These situations are few, and as such, we are most often able to increase the safety of transfusion medicine by performing blood typing test(s) before administration of blood products.

Blood typing relies heavily on the visible reaction that occurs when blood agglutinates. Agglutination is the process in which RBCs come together and stick to each other in a nonspecific pattern (Fig. 11.1). The cells join in random order and collect in a clump shaped like a cluster of grapes (Mathews 2006). The agglutination pattern is not to be confused with rouleaux, a grouping of cells comparable with a stack of coins.

A common method of blood typing uses a small sample of blood and a pretreated card with reagent-filled windows. There is an appreciable reaction with the reagent in one of the test windows that allows the operator to determine the animal's blood type. Animals with diseases involving autoagglutination present an interesting dilemma for blood typing. Because their blood is already agglutinating, it cannot be certain that the reaction noted on a test card is actually due to reaction with the reagent rather than autoagglutination due to the patient's disease. In dogs with a confounding test result, it is safer to assume that the patient is negative for RBC membrane antigens that are common in the species and to transfuse with a blood from an A− donor. In cats, it is difficult to follow the same reasoning, but if no other options are available and the patient is a domestic short- or long-haired cat, it is likely that the cat is type A. Further testing is required before transfusing auto agglutinating patients due to the difficulty encountered in interpreting agglutination on blood typing cards.

Canine blood typing

Blood typing cards are a user-friendly point-of-care testing method used to differentiate DEA 1.1 positive dogs from DEA 1.1 negative dogs. The cards only screen for antigens at the 1.1 location and can only be used as a preliminary testing method for determining the blood type of a canine patient. A dog that screens as A− on a typing card still has the

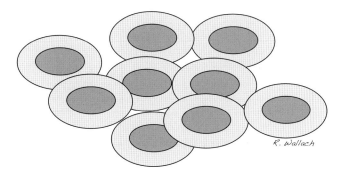

Agglutinated RBC's

Figure 11.1. Red blood cells stick together in this arrangement in a process called agglutination. Illustration by Rachel Wallach.

potential to be positive for the DEA 1.2 location. Because the card does not screen for this location on the RBC membrane, it is not a foolproof way of ensuring that the dog is truly A−. If the recipient's blood type is in question and A− blood is available, it is considered safe practice to administer an A− transfusion to the patient even with the potential for the patient to be antigen positive at DEA 1.2. Conversely, if it is the donor's blood that tests negative on the typing card, further testing is still required in case the donor is positive for DEA 1.2. Administering blood that types negative on preliminary screening to an A− recipient can have serious consequences if the donor is in fact DEA 1.2 positive.

Use of the blood typing cards is straightforward, and the instructions provided are clear and easy to follow. In general, canine typing cards involve a window to test for autoagglutination, two control windows, and a test window. The reagents in the windows are reconstituted with the diluent provided. Once reconstituted, a drop of patient blood is applied and the liquids are stirred with individual stirrers provided in the package. The card is then rocked and the tester observes for signs of agglutination. Agglutination should appear in the 1.1 positive control window. If the patient test window shows agglutination, the patient is DEA 1.1 positive. If the patient test window shows no reaction, the patient is DEA 1.1 negative.

Further testing is required to identify blood types specifically in blood donors. It is beneficial to identify whether canine donors and recipients are positive or negative for the *Dal* antigen as well. This process is not possible using the test cards.

It is important to remember that the efficacy of the typing cards may be compromised in patients with autoagglutination or marked anemia.

Blood typing can also be performed using a technique that involves columns of gel rather than flat cards. Small tubes are used to house the reagents. At the lower end of the tubes, the gel acts as a filter and only the RBCs that are not agglutinated pass through the filter and congregate at the bottom. The cells that agglutinate are easily observed suspended in the gel medium at the lower end of the tube. Benefits associated with this method of blood typing include easy interpretation and preservation of the reacted cells in the gel. The stability provided by the gel allows the agglutinated cells to be reviewed for a longer period of time. To date, the results obtained from the gel method are largely compatible with those obtained from the card method (Tocci and Ewing 2009).

Feline blood typing

Feline blood typing is carried out in much the same manner as canine. Species-specific blood typing cards are used and the method is similar (Fig. 11.2).

Feline typing cards have three windows coated with dried reagent. The first window is used to verify that the patient is not autoagglutinating. Its test is completed before initiating the rest of the typing procedure. The second and third windows determine blood type.

The reagent windows are reconstituted using the diluents provided with the test. A drop of the patient's blood is then incorporated onto each window and mixed well with reagent. A clean stirring utensil is used for each window. If agglutination is apparent in the reagent window for type A, then the cat is blood type A. If the agglutination is apparent in window B, the cat is blood type B. If there appears to be agglutination in both windows, the cat is type AB.

Blood typing cards for cats provide a true blood type for each animal screened. In contrast to the typing cards for dogs, which only type the location for DEA 1.1 and may falsely identify a 1.2 positive donor as A−, the feline typing cards firmly ascertain whether the cat is type A, B, or AB.

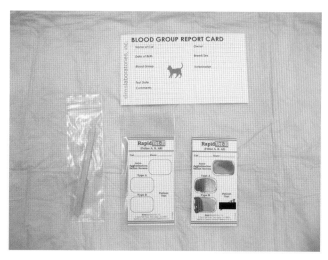

Figure 11.2. Blood typing cards are a convenient way to determine feline blood types. Tests can be used at cage side and are a cost-effective way of increasing the safety of feline blood transfusions.

Determining Donor Recipient Compatibility

In addition to blood typing donors and recipients, the safety of blood transfusions can be increased by determining whether the donor blood is compatible with the recipient blood. It is possible for the recipient to react to the donor's blood despite having the same blood type. This is in part due to the existence of RBC membrane antigens that are not yet recognized and for which no cage-side screening or typing yet exists.

Major crossmatch

The major crossmatch is performed to determine the compatibility of donor blood and recipient blood. Proper completion of the cross match that yields no evidence of agglutination contributes to safe administration of blood transfusions. A cross match can significantly reduce the chances of a hemolytic reaction in the recipient.

In this procedure RBCs from the donor are washed and then mixed with serum from the recipient. Evidence of agglutination confirms that the donor blood is *not compatible* with the recipient and should not be used for a transfusion in this patient. If there is no suggestion of agglutination, the donor and recipient are compatible and the blood can be used for transfusion. It is important to recall that despite a compatible result from the cross-match screening, a recipient may still have a reaction to the transfusion that results in red cell destruction.

Agglutination confirms that the recipient has a preformed antibody to the donor's RBCs. The cross match does not determine whether this antibody was present from birth or whether due to sensitization via previous transfusion of blood products. In either case, the cross match gives a visibly appreciable result that rules out the donor sample tested.

Because the cross match relies heavily on agglutination as a marker of incompatibility, the test is less reliable in patients whose disease involves autoagglutination. Patients suffering from immune-mediated hemolytic anemia are often autoagglutinating. A cross match performed for one of these patients will likely yield a positive result due to the ongoing destruction of RBCs that is a part of the disease. Cross matches may not be a valuable pretransfusion screening test for these patients.

Minor cross match

The minor cross match evaluates the compatibility between the donor's plasma and the recipient's blood. The recipient's RBCs are washed and mixed with donor plasma. After a period of incubation (procedure is similar to that of major cross match), the sample is inspected for evidence of agglutination. If agglutination is documented, the transfusion would not be compatible with the recipient.

Blood Collection

Operating procedures vary from practice to practice. The following methods can be used as a guideline for the processes involved for safe and smooth blood donations. These are by no means the only methods available.

Canine blood donation

The goal of the technician should be to make the donation process as smooth, stress free, and comfortable as possible for the donor. The technician should use any opportunity to decrease the amount of anxiety that a donor may experience. If donors have been selected according to recommended guidelines, most will have a personality that is not highly stressed to begin with.

A standard canine blood donation involves removal of approximately 450 mL of WB. A guideline of 16 to 18 mL of blood per kilogram of body weight should maintain the collection within safe parameters (Ogg 2001). Dogs donating through a blood donor program can typically donate blood every 3 to 4 weeks.

A physical examination should be performed before every donation. Accurate record-keeping is essential. Once the physical examination is completed, a small blood sample may be obtained from a peripheral vessel to evaluate the donor's packed cell volume (PCV). Dogs with PCVs less than 40% should not be used for donation (Giger 2010). A stick blood urea nitrogen (BUN) should also be included in the precollection examination.

The technician should record which jugular vein is used and which peripheral vein is catheterized (if any) for each collection. The same vessel(s) should not be used in consecutive collections but should be alternated at each visit. Once the jugular vein has been selected, the hair is clipped and topical anaesthetic cream is applied to the skin. The cream should be applied approximately 30 to 60 minutes before collection; with 60 minutes the goal. Covering the shaved area may increase the efficacy of the cream.

Sedation is required for some canine donors. Practices that choose to place peripheral intravenous (IV) catheters can administer sedation by this route. Otherwise, the technician should choose a route that involves as little time and discomfort as possible. A narcotic analgesic is a sound choice for sedation for the canine blood donor. Low doses of butorphanol (0.2 mg/kg) or hydromorphone (0.05 mg/kg) offer the added benefit of

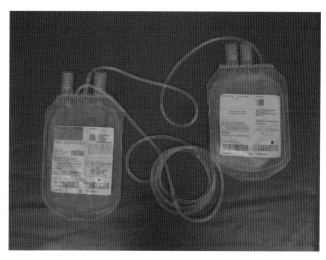

Figure 11.3. Closed systems are used for canine blood collection. The double bag allows for separation of components.

analgesia as well as sedation. Other sedatives may be used, but the technician should avoid administering medications that cause hypotension because they can complicate the collection and potentially compromise the donor's safety. Glycopyrrolate is helpful to reduce the secretion of saliva in the sedated animal (0.005 mg/kg) (Mathews 2006).

A three-stage surgical preparation of the shaved area over the jugular vein is used to rid the skin of dirt and debris. The dog is then placed in lateral recumbency. The person restraining the dog is also responsible for occluding or "holding off" the jugular vein. The technician places the large gauge needle into the jugular vein and holds it in place throughout the collection process. Care should be taken not to move the needle back and forth or in and out of the vessel. Trauma to the vascular lining can lead to complications after collection.

The average volume of WB collected from a canine donor is 450 mL per donation. Collection systems are available that are preloaded with anticoagulant (Fig. 11.3). These are closed systems where the needle is attached to tubing that leads directly into the collection bag. The bag is weighed before, during, and after the donation to measure the volume of collected blood. A vacuum tube can be placed on a small scale so that once the suction is activated and the blood flows into the bag, the scale continuously measures the volume in the bag. Once the goal volume is reached, the suction is turned off and the needle is withdrawn from the donor's jugular vein.

Blood should be directed out of the lines and into the bag after collection. The WB is mixed with the anticoagulant and a small volume can be allowed to flow back into the tubing. A clamp is then applied to the line close to the bag to ensure that no further blood product leaks out of the bag and into the line. Additional clamps can be placed at intervals along the line to provide small volumes of blood that can be used for PCV evaluation and other screening tests. The remainder of the collection line and the needle should be disposed of appropriately.

Pressure should be applied to the donor's neck at the venipuncture site immediately upon termination of collection. Pressure should remain for several minutes to curtail hematoma formation. The donor's neck can be wrapped temporarily as an additional precaution.

The donor should remain in the care of the technician until time of discharge. A quiet and comfortable housing situation that facilitates frequent post-donation monitoring is ideal. The donor should be well rewarded for the contribution.

Feline blood donation

Each hospital must decide on a standard operating procedure that is safe for feline donors in their care. One of the main variables encountered with feline donation in different clinical settings is the use of general anaesthesia via inhalant agents versus heavy sedation using injectable agents. Either procedure is acceptable as long as safety precautions and patient well-being supersede other goals.

Each feline blood donor should be examined before the blood collection. Temperature, pulse, and respiration (TPR) should be recorded in the animal's patient record, as well as body weight on the day of the donation. A small amount of blood work is recommended before donation. The sample may be obtained from a peripheral vessel or from a peripherally placed IV catheter prior to injection of any medication or flush. In some blood donor programs, peripheral catheters are not placed until the feline donor has been sedated or anaesthetized. Much of this depends on the personality and approachability of the cat. Moderate sedation can be achieved via intramuscular or subcutaneous (SC) injection, which often facilitates placement of an IV catheter.

Blood collected from the IV catheter or the peripheral vein should be used to evaluate PCV/total solids (TS) and stick BUN as a minimum database. Feline blood donation should not be carried out if the donor's PCV is less than 28% (Mathews 2006).

If the protocol includes sedation but not anaesthesia, the donor should receive oxygen via face mask once sedation has taken effect. Donors that are intubated and anaesthetized receive oxygen via endotracheal tube with their anaesthetic gas. The cat's eyes should be lubricated with ophthalmic ointment. At the Ontario Veterinary College feline donors receive 90 mL of SC fluid before donation. Most often this is 0.9% sodium chloride.

A generous area around the jugular vein is clipped and surgically prepared (Fig. 11.4). The phlebotomist must have clean hands and should observe strict aseptic technique when handling the prepared area of the jugular vein and the butterfly needle. Wearing gloves is advisable; however it may add an element of difficulty when palpating the jugular vein.

Blood is collected into a 60-mL syringe that has been preloaded with 8 mL of anticoagulant (Fig. 11.5). Venipuncture is best achieved using a butterfly needle (19G works well), and the tubing is subsequently attached to the syringe once the needle is seated in the vessel. A slow steady negative pressure is applied to the syringe to withdraw blood. The syringe should be inverted often throughout the donation to ensure that the anticoagulant mixes well with the blood.

Monitoring the patient is paramount to safe blood donation. Heart rate, respiratory rate, and blood pressure should be evaluated frequently. It is common for the systolic blood pressure to drop quite low once the collection reaches the point at which 40 mL have been withdrawn. The technician must use judgment with respect to whether or not it is safe to continue the collection. In most cases, the blood continues to flow into the syringe without too much difficulty and the collection can be completed without interruption. In the event that the blood draw becomes more challenging and less blood is flowing into the syringe despite continuous negative pressure, the collection should be

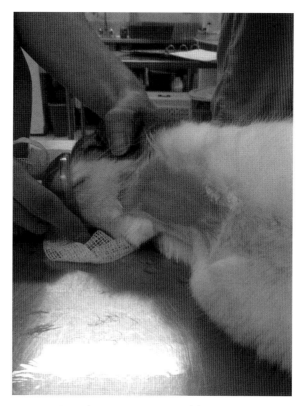

Figure 11.4. A three-stage prep is used on a generous area of the jugular vein of feline donors.

terminated immediately and the patient should be fluid resuscitated. In uncomplicated donations, the donor receives the remainder of the fluid IV after collection (60 mL 0.9% NaCl). It is important to deliver these fluids slowly. Fast delivery of IV fluids post donation expands the intravascular space very quickly. Bradycardia and pulmonary edema are possible undesirable side effects (Ogg 2001).

As the cat recovers from the sedation or anaesthesia, the animal should be visible to the technician at all times. Frequent evaluation of temperature, heart rate, and blood pressure are recommended during the recovery phase. Hypovolemia is still a possible side effect in spite of the replacement fluid therapy that the donor received pre and post donation. The cat should be alert, ambulatory, normothermic, normotensive, and eating well before discharge from the hospital.

Processing Blood and Creating Components

Anticoagulant is mixed with WB to render it useful post collection. Two- and three-bag blood collection systems come preloaded with the anticoagulant citrate phosphate dextrose adenine (CPDA). The citrate component is an anticoagulant that prevents blood clots from forming once the blood is mixed in the collection bag and line. The phosphate acts as a buffer for the products created as a result of RBC metabolism. The dextrose

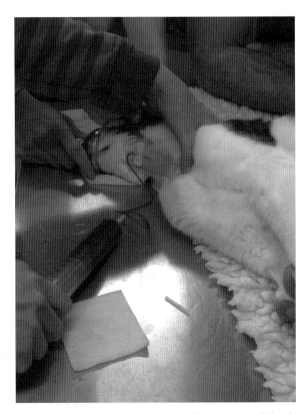

Figure 11.5. Feline blood collection involves a slow and steady aspiration of blood into a prepared syringe.

and the adenine are included in the bags to preserve the cells in a healthy state (Lucas et al. 2004).

Acid, citrate, and dextrose (ACD) is another anticoagulant used for blood donation. Blood mixed with ACD typically has a shelf life of 21 days (Green 2002). Adsol and Nutricel are RBC preservatives. These products can be added to PRBCs to lengthen the safe window for use of the component. They typically extend shelf life to approximately 30 to 35 days (Lucas et al. 2004).

Fresh whole blood

Blood removed from a donor and not processed in any way other than mixed with anticoagulant is referred to as fresh whole blood (FWB). As such, it contains all of the blood components: RBCs, white blood cells (WBCs), coagulation factors, platelets, and plasma proteins. FWB should be administered to the recipient within 4 to 6 hours of collection to conserve as many beneficial characteristics as possible (Chiaramonte 2004). For example, coagulation factors and platelets lose their effectiveness as more time elapses between collection and administration.

FWB not used for transfusion within 6 to 8 hours of collection can be saved and used as stored WB, which is refrigerated at 4°C and is usable for up to 35 days if mixed with CPDA 1 (Figs. 11.6 and 11.7).

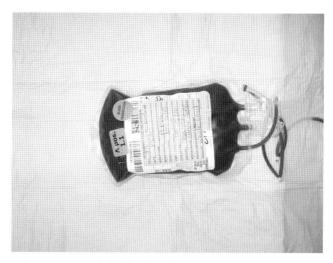

Figure 11.6. A unit of canine stored whole blood. Each unit measures approximately 450 mL. Note the labeling on the bag. Clear identification is necessary to contribute to the safety of transfusion medicine. The circular blood transfusion sticker may be removed and placed in the recipient's file to indicate that the patient has received blood products.

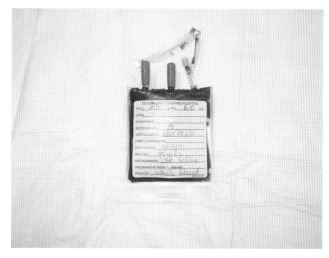

Figure 11.7. Feline whole blood is stored in smaller bags. The bags can be spiked or the blood can be removed and transfused via syringe on a syringe driver.

Indications

FWB is the product of choice in a number of clinical situations. Patients that have undergone trauma resulting in massive acute hemorrhage use not only the red cell oxygen-carrying capacity in WB but also the coagulation factors. Similarly, a patient with a coagulation disorder may also benefit from a transfusion of FWB. Anemia arising from loss of WB rather than simply RBC destruction may be treated with FWB transfusion to replenish the cellular component as well as the plasma component of the animal's intravascular body water. A transfusion of 20 mL/kg of FWB can raise a patient's PCV by approximately 10% (Chiaramonte 2004).

WB contains the same RBCs and plasma proteins as FWB, but many of its coagulation factors are no longer functional. Factors dependent on vitamin K remain active in WB, but factor VIII, von Willebrand factor, and factor V are inactive. For this reason, WB is not the product of choice in patients that require coagulation factors or platelets because these are rendered inactive by refrigeration and as time elapses after collection.

Packed red blood cells and fresh frozen plasma

Fresh frozen plasma (FFP) and PRBCs are prepared simultaneously in most blood banking programs (Figs. 11.8, 11.9, and 11.10). FWB is centrifuged at roughly 4000 rotations per minute for between 10 and 15 minutes (Chiaramonte 2004; Lucas et al.

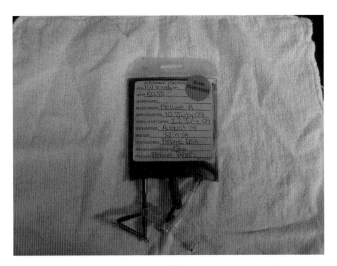

Figure 11.8.   One unit of feline packed RBCs. Whole blood can be separated into components. Due to the small volume removed from feline donors, feline blood is separated into PRBCs and FFP only.

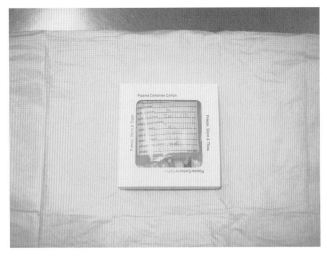

Figure 11.9.   A unit of feline FFP. FFP is stored in boxes as well as bags. The box is an additional means of protecting the frozen product.

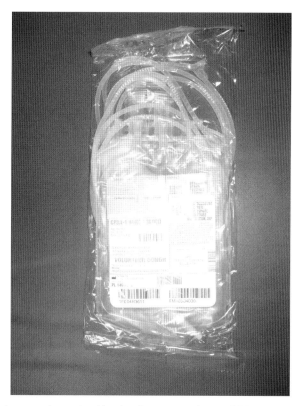

Figure 11.10. Closed systems for canine blood collection are also available with three bags.

2004). Opinions vary regarding the appropriate temperature at which the blood should be centrifuged. Most recommend storing and centrifuging FWB at 4°C if it is to be used for PRBC and FFP products. Once the FWB is centrifuged, the plasma is separated from the RBCs. This is facilitated through the use of the two- or three-bag collection system whereby the products are maintained in a closed system and sterility is preserved via transfer of products through sterile lines between bags.

PRBCs can be stored at 4°C for up to 20 days unless they have been prepared with a preservative. Preservative solutions allow PRBCs to be refrigerated for up to 35 days (Gibson 2007).

Plasma is considered FFP if it is separated and frozen no more than 8 hours after collection from the donor. (Note: Plasma must be frozen by 8 hours, not beginning to freeze by 8 hours.) If these guidelines are followed, the FFP contains coagulation factors and plasma proteins that are useful in many situations. FFP is stored at −20° for up to 1 year.

Fresh plasma (FP) is the product name for FFP that has been thawed, not used, and refrozen, that has not been used within 1 year of freezing, or that has not been separated within 6 hours of collection from donor (Gibson 2007).

Indications

PRBCs are similar to WB in that they can provide oxygen-carrying capacity to anemic animals. One of the benefits of PRBCs is that the volume of the transfusion is far smaller than that of a WB transfusion despite a similar number of RBCs. The concentration of

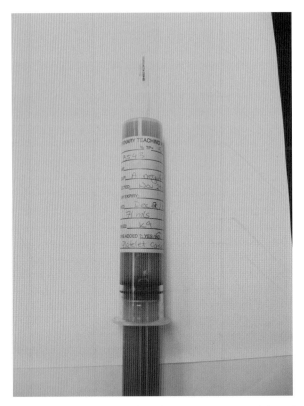

Figure 11.11. Patients actively bleeding due to thrombocytopenia are candidates for platelet concentrate transfusions.

the PRBCs is much higher, and the PCV of a unit of PRBCs generally runs between 70% and 80% (Green 2002). PRBCs are an appropriate choice of blood product for patients with anemia that do not have an associated hypovolemia. Animals that are at risk for or extremely sensitive to volume overload should be transfused with PRBCs over FWB to reduce the volume of fluid delivered. The technician can expect to see a 1% increase in PCV for every milliliter of PRBC per kilogram that a patient receives (Mathews 2006).

FFP is indicated in animals that have coagulation defects whether these are inherited or acquired. Examples of inherited coagulopathies that may respond to FFP transfusions include vitamin K deficiency, von Willebrand factor deficiency, and hemophilia. Acquired coagulopathies that may be treated with FFP include warfarin toxicity, disseminated intravascular coagulation, and liver failure.

Platelet-rich plasma and platelet concentrate

Platelets are fragile elements of FWB. They require special handling to preserve their function. The decision to make platelet products must be made before blood donation. The blood must be collected into a latex-free, heparin-free system and must not be refrigerated at any time prior to separation of components (Fig. 11.11).

To create PRP, FWB is centrifuged at a lower speed and for a shorter time than for FFP and PRBCs. The plasma supernatant is separated as with other plasma components, but due to the special centrifugation, it contains a higher concentration of platelets. If platelet concentrate (PC) is desired, the PRP is centrifuged again. The PRP should be in a bag that is part of a closed system with a second empty bag. Once the PRP has been spun, the top layer of plasma is moved into the second bag. This second bag can then be frozen and is considered to be FFP. The small volume left in the initial bag should be approximately 50 mL and is the component referred to as PC (Green 2002).

Ideally, the platelet products are used promptly after separation. If this is not possible, they can be maintained at room temperature for up to 5 days. The products should be kept on a rocker that sustains continuous gentle motion.

If platelet products are derived using an open collection system, sterility is not as reliable. PRP and PC are not refrigerated and as such should be used within 4 hours of collection if an open system is used during production (Gibson 2007).

Platelet harvesting by apheresis is a less common but very effective practice. Blood is removed from a donor and processed in a closed system before being returned to the donor. As the blood is removed, it is mixed with anticoagulant as it passes through the apheresis circuit. The components are then separated via centrifugation. This process yields PC, and the plasma and RBCs return to the donor. Benefits of this system include a higher platelet count in the PC, fewer stray RBCs and WBCs in the PC product, and a decrease in immune reaction in the recipient (Callan et al. 2009). Hypocalcemia is a possible side effect for the donor due to the use of citrate anticoagulant in the blood that is returned after apheresis.

Indications

Blood components that target high platelet numbers are reserved for very specific situations (Fig. 11.12). Because the amount of platelets obtained from one unit of PRP or PC is still relatively small, a transfusion of these components might make little difference to a thrombocytopenic animal. In immune thrombocytopenia purpura (ITP) patients, the infused platelets are also attacked by the immune system and destroyed. The use of PRP or PC is controversial for these patients. In some clinical settings it is feasible to load platelets with products that combat the immune-mediated disease that seeks to destroy them. In this situation it may be appropriate to provide an ITP patient with a PRP or PC transfusion (Mathews 2006). Patients with life-threatening active bleeding due to platelet defects or disorders (thrombocytopenia or thrombocytopathia) may also require platelet transfusion (Callan et al. 2009).

Cryoprecipitate

Cryoprecipitate (Cryo) is a component derived from FFP. The plasma is slowly thawed and then centrifuged while there is still a small amount of frozen plasma in the bag. The centrifuge is set for 5000 rpm for 5 minutes. Ideally, the temperature in the centrifuge should be close to 4°C. A white precipitate forms after the FFP is spun, which is separated from the liquid plasma. The supernatant is still a functional blood product because it is rich in clotting factors, albumin, and globulin. The substance remaining in the bag is the Cryo, and it contains high concentrations of von Willebrand factor, factors VIII, XI, and XII, and fibrinogen.

Both the C and the C supernatant must be refrozen after separation. They may be stored for 1 year at −20°C (Chiaramonte 2004).

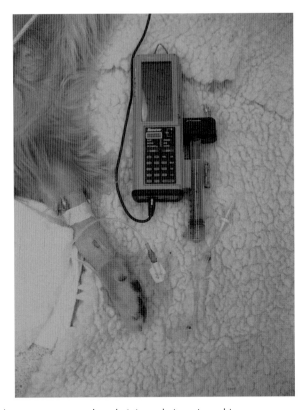

Figure 11.12.   Platelet concentrate can be administered via syringe driver.

Indications

Cryo transfusions are reserved for patients with von Willebrand factor deficiency or hemophilia A (factor VIII dysfunction). Cryosupernatant may be used in hypoprotein-emic patients or for patients with coagulopathies not specifically related to factors remaining in cryoprecipitate.

Blood Transfusions

The decision to deliver blood products to a hospitalized patient is one that requires much thought and planning. Transfusions, although potentially lifesaving, are also associated with immune reactions that can be life threatening to the recipient. Precautions are taken to markedly improve the margin of transfusion safety, but it is impossible to completely eliminate the risks associated with the administration of blood products.

Before administering a blood transfusion it is necessary to determine which blood product is most suitable for each situation. The clinician should consider the primary reason for the transfusion. For example,

■ Does the patient require oxygen-carrying capacity?
■ Does the patient require clotting factors?

- Has the patient received previous transfusion(s) of blood products?
- Is the patient normovolemic or hypovolemic?
- If the patient is anemic, is the condition acute or chronic?

Answering these types of questions facilitates selection of a blood component that is appropriate for individual patients. Decisions regarding blood product selection are also influenced by which components are available. An acutely anemic animal can benefit from a PRBC transfusion or a WB transfusion, but the clinical situation may be such that only one of the two products is available. In contrast, a hospital that has its own blood donor program may be flush with blood products and have the choice of all of the different components. The technician must consider how to best use their resources regardless of the ease with which she or he can access blood products.

Setting up a transfusion

Blood products are delivered through special blood administration sets that house a filter within the line. In most systems the filter is found in the drip chamber. The blood flows out of the bag, through the spike, and into the filter so that any small clots that might have formed during storage are trapped by the filter and not delivered to the patient. Pore sizes of 170 μm to 270 μm are recommended for blood component therapy. Smaller sizes are available, but these are prone to obstructing and also can filter out platelets (Giger 2010). Platelet products must only be delivered through nonlatex transfusion sets.

Once the blood component has been selected, the bag should be visually examined to confirm the absence of large blood clots. Bags should also be inspected for any possible breach of sterility because frozen products can easily sustain cracks to the bag before thawing. The technician should confirm that the product chosen is the correct component, the correct blood type, and that its use is taking place before its expiration date.

Frozen products may be thawed using a gentle warm water bath or in a commercial plasma thawer. Care must be taken not to overheat the product because excessive warmth can encourage growth of bacteria that may be present. Overheating blood products also destroys clotting factors and can denature plasma proteins.

The line delivering the blood product can be piggybacked onto the main fluid infusion set. It is advisable to connect the blood administration line to a port close to the animal, particularly if the flow of fluids with or without blood products is very slow. There is no need for the blood product to sit in the fluid line for any longer than necessary. As hospitals move toward needleless practice, it becomes easier to piggyback lines using Luer lock ports.

Monitoring the transfusion

The patient must be examined before beginning the transfusion. Pretransfusion temperature and pulse is recorded on the patient's chart. Blood products are delivered slowly for the first few minutes so that the technician may observe any sign that the patient is reacting to the infusion. A small dose known as the *test dose* is administered after the TPR. Test doses are administered at a rate of 0.25 mL/kg per hour. At the Ontario Veterinary College Teaching Hospital, we administer the test dose over 15 minutes. For example, to determine a test dose for a 48-kg dog:

$$Rate = 0.25 \text{ mL/kg per hour} = 0.25 \text{ mL} \times 48 \text{ kg} = 12 \text{ mL/h}$$

$$\text{Volume to be infused (over 15 minutes)} = 12 \text{ mL/60 min: x mL/15 min}$$

$$\text{cross-multiply} = 12 \text{ mL} \times 15 \text{ min} \div 60 \text{ min} = 3 \text{ mL}$$

Thus the 48-kg dog will receive a volume of 3 mL of blood over 15 minutes at a rate of 12 mL/h for its test dose.

Once the test dose has been administered, the TPR is repeated and recorded on the chart. Increases in any of the parameters of the TPR are concerning and may be reflective of incompatibility of the blood product. A second test dose may be administered if there is any doubt that the patient may be staging a reaction to the blood transfusion. After the second test dose is administered, another TPR is performed. Discretion is necessary because in some cases it may not be appropriate to repeat the test dose. If the animal is displaying any other signs of transfusion reaction after the first or second test dose, the transfusion should be terminated and the clinician should be consulted. If there are no further changes to the animal's condition, it may be possible to continue the transfusion. The clinician should be alerted regarding any change in the patient's condition associated with infusion of a blood component. In some cases, it may be appropriate to treat the animal with diphenhydramine (0.5 mg/kg) either prophylactically, before the start of the infusion, or after the test dose if there are mild concerns (Chiaramonte 2004).

The transfusion may continue at a higher flow rate if there are no changes to the animal's TPR or condition during the test dose. It is recommended that blood components be delivered within 4 hours of being spiked. Extending the transfusion time increases the chances for contamination. A rate for the transfusion can be determined by dividing the volume of the bag by 4 hours, which results in a rate in milliliters per hour. For the average canine unit of blood, the calculation would be as follows:

- 450 mL ÷ 4 h = 112.5 mL/h
- The flow rate can be rounded up or down to 113 or 112 mL/h, respectively

Transfusions may need to be administered over longer periods of time for patients that have concurrent heart disease or that may be compromised by faster infusions.

Patients should be closely monitored throughout their blood product transfusion. Close monitoring should continue for the 24-hour period following transfusion as well because delayed transfusion reactions are possible.

The recipient's packed cell volume should be measured 1 to 2 hours posttransfusion to determine the impact of the blood product. This evaluation is not mandatory if the transfusion did not include RBCs.

Transfusion Reactions

Transfusion reactions are a potential threat that cannot be entirely eliminated. Several different types of transfusion reactions are documented in recipients. These vary with regard to the cells that trigger the reactions, the timing of the onset of the reaction, and the clinical signs witnessed in the recipient. Transfusion reactions are categorized into four groups that are highlighted here.

Immune responses staged against antigens found on RBC membranes are the most common transfusion reactions. In general, these reactions occur soon after delivery of the blood product. The RBCs are destroyed within the vascular space (acute haemolytic reaction) due to their foreign antigens (Chiaramonte 2004). This type of reaction falls under the category of *acute immunologic reactions*. The technician may appreciate increases in temperature, heart rate, and respiratory rate with a concurrent decrease in blood pressure. The patient's urine may develop a brownish tinge due to hemoglobinuria, a by-product of the intravascular hemolysis.

The recipient may also react to donor WBCs and platelets found in the transfused component. In this type of reaction, the patient develops a mild fever. The RBCs are not destroyed and there is no hemolysis. This reaction, known as an acute febrile non-hemolytic reaction, is observed within half an hour of the start of the transfusion (Chiaramonte 2004). Clinical signs of this reaction can be evident for close to a full day. It is also classified as an *acute immunologic reaction.*

Acute nonimmunologic reactions include a wide range of clinical signs and physiologic changes that take place during or shortly after the transfusion. These include electrolyte defects, volume overload, contamination of blood products, and damage sustained by blood component due to mishandling (Hohenhaus 2006).

Immunologic and non-immunologic transfusion reactions can also be delayed. The *delayed immunologic reactions* that occur posttransfusion are a result of antibodies that develop in response to foreign antigens. Preventive measures such as cross matching and blood typing do not prevent this type of reaction. Clinical signs such as purpura are associated with these reactions and can manifest 1 week posttransfusion and last for up to 2 months (Chiaramonte 2004). *Purpura* is a term that describes small reddish purple markings that appear on the patient's skin. The recipient's allo-antibodies attack and destroy the patient's platelets, potentially leading to thrombocytopenia. The red or purple marks, similar to but larger than petechiae, are areas of bleeding underneath the animal's skin. *Delayed nonimmunologic transfusion reactions* are the result of disease transmission through transfused blood components. Blood from a donor with a viral infection exposes the recipient to the disease. Development of that disease in the recipient is an example of a delayed nonimmunologic reaction (Hohenhaus 2006).

The technician must be diligent in the monitoring routine during administration of blood products. Early recognition of clinical signs associated with acute transfusion reactions is imperative. Cessation of the transfusion is warranted until the clinician can be notified of the changes in patient status. Thorough evaluation of the patient and consideration of individual patient needs and circumstances must be undertaken by the medical team before institution of further treatments.

Autotransfusion

Autotransfusion is the process by which an animal is given a transfusion of WB that has been collected from a hemorrhage into one of its body cavities (abdomen or thorax) (Figs. 11.13, 11.14, and 11.15). This type of transfusion, like any other, has associated risks and benefits. Ideally, WB, FWB, or PRBCs should be available for a patient experiencing a life-threatening hemorrhage.

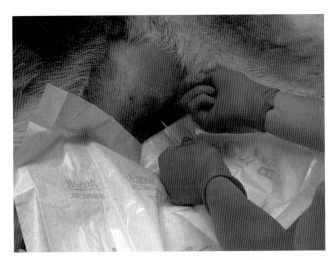

Figure 11.13. Sterile technique is observed while inserting a large-bore catheter into the peritoneal cavity. This patient has a hemoabdomen. Blood is collected for potential autotranfusion.

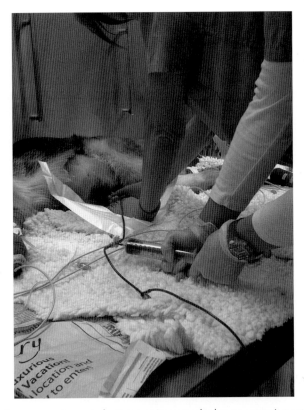

Figure 11.14. Negative pressure is created using a syringe attached to an extension set attached to the catheter. A three-way stopcock facilitates transfer of the blood into a collection system.

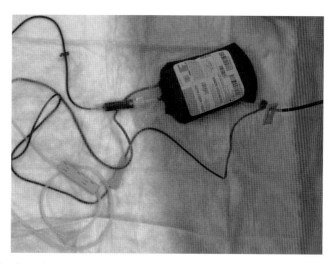

Figure 11.15. Blood is infused into the collection bag and can be stored for the patient from whom it was collected. Alternatively, it can be immediately transfused into the patient. A typical blood transfusion set is recommended due to the presence of an inline filter.

The patient's blood is removed via large-bore catheter into a syringe and, where possible, it can be transferred through a closed system into an anticoagulant loaded collection bag by way of a three-way stopcock. An inline filter is required for administration of collected blood back into the patient's vasculature.

Transfusing the patient's own blood back into circulation has the benefit of providing body temperature appropriately typed blood product at little cost to the client. In contrast, autotransfusion is plagued by multiple opportunities for the blood to become contaminated.

Autotransfusion is not an acceptable mode of blood transfusion in patients whose hemorrhage is associated with a neoplastic process. For example, a dog that has a hemoabdomen due to rupture of a splenic mass is not a candidate for autotransfusion. It is possible that some of the blood contained within the abdominal cavity has been present for an unknown length of time (associated with previous subclinical episodes of bleeding), and as such it is not suitable for reintroduction to circulation. Furthermore, the blood within the abdominal cavity is the product of a ruptured tumor and is thought to contain cancer cells. Autotransfusion of blood potentially containing neoplastic cells is counterintuitive.

Chapter Summary

Transfusion medicine is a valuable tool in emergency and critical care medicine. Blood can be collected from donor animals and divided into sections called components. Blood components include packed red blood cells, plasma, platelet-rich plasma, platelet concentrate, and cryoprecipitate. Each of these components can be transfused to a recipient in need of specific hematologic support providing the product is of the same blood type as the recipient's. Blood typing and cross matching are tests that identify an animal's blood type and determine the compatibility of donor/recipient blood samples, respectively. Identifying a patient's blood type and assessing compatibility of samples contribute to safe transfusion of blood products. Despite cautious screening, blood transfusion reactions are still possible and can be life threatening.

Autotransfusion is the process by which an animal's blood is removed from a body cavity posthemorrhage, mixed with anticoagulant, and given back to the patient. This process also has associated risks and should be reserved for the extreme situations where no other blood product is available.

Review Questions

1. What are the ideal age and weight requirements for canine blood donors?
2. What are the ideal age and weight requirements for feline blood donors?
3. Of the dog erythrocyte antigens, which locations are the most clinically relevant with regard to transfusion medicine?
4. Cats also have their own blood types. Name the three feline blood types and identify which of these is the most common feline blood type in the United States and Canada.
5. Blood collected from a canine donor is collected into a closed system preloaded with which additive?
6. What is the purpose of this additive?
7. Which blood product would be most appropriate for administration to a patient that is severely anemic but is not hypovolemic and has a total protein within normal limits?
8. Which vital signs are recorded and compared before and after a patient receives a test dose of a blood product?
9. What is autotransfusion?

Answers to the review questions can be found on page 225 in the Appendix. The review questions are also available for download on a companion website at www.wiley.com/go/donohoenursing.

Further Reading

Blais, M. et al. 2002. Canine *Dal* blood type: a red cell antigen lacking in some dalmations. *J Vet Intern Med* 21:281–286.

Callan, M., E. Appleman, and B. Sachais. 2009. Canine platelet transfusions. *J Vet Emerg Crit Care* 19:401–415.

Chiaramonte, D. 2004. Blood-component therapy: selection, administration and monitoring. *Clin Tech Small Anim Pract* 19:63–67.

Gibson, G. 2007. Storing blood: what can I do and how? British Small Animal Veterinary Congress Proceedings; Birmingham.

Giger, U. 2010. Transfusion medicine—do's and don'ts. Proceedings World Small Animal Veterinary Association Congress; Switzerland.

Green, M. 2002. Transfusion medicine. In W. E. Wingfield, ed. *The ICU Book*, 189–202. Jackson, WY: Teton NewMedia.

Hohenhaus, A. 2006. Blood transfusion and blood substitutes. In S. DiBartola, ed. *Fluid, Electrolyte, and Acid-Base Disorders in Small Animal Practice*, 567–581. St. Louis: Elsevier.

Lucas, R., K. Lentz, and A. Hale. 2004. Collection and preparation of blood products. *Clin Tech Small Anim Pract* 19:55–62.

Mathews, K. 2006. Transfusion of blood products. In *Veterinary Emergency and Critical Care Manual*, 667–681. Guelph, Ontario, Canada: LifeLearn.

Ogg, A. A. 2001. Practical blood transfusion. In M. J. Day, A. Mackin, and J. Littlewood, eds. *BSAVA Manual of Canine and Feline Haematology and Transfusion Medicine*, Chapter 15. Quedgeley, Gloucester, UK: British Small Animal Veterinary Association.

Prittie, J. 2010. Controversies related to red blood cell transfusion in critically ill patients. *J Vet Emerg Crit Care* 20:167–176.

Rozanski, E., and A. de Laforcade. 2004. Transfusion medicine in veterinary emergency and critical care medicine. *Clin Tech Small Anim Pract* 19:83–87.

Snow, S., A. Jutkowitz, and A. Brown. 2010. Trends in plasma transfusion at a veterinary teaching hospital: 308 patients (1996–1998 and 2006–2008). *J Vet Emerg Crit Care* 20:441–445.

Tocci, L., and P. Ewing. 2009. Increasing patient safety in veterinary transfusion medicine: an overview of pretransfusion testing. *J Vet Emerg Crit Care* 19:66–73.

Weinstein, N. 2007. A newly recognized blood group in domestic shorthair cats: the Mik red cell antigen. *J Vet Intern Med* 21:287–292.

Appendix
Answers to Review Questions

Chapter 1

1. 60%
2. Higher. Approximately 80% of body weight is water in neonates.
3. Approximately 5%
4. Osmosis is the process by which water passes through a semipermeable membrane into an area of higher solute concentration.
5. Sodium and chloride are the primary electrolytes found in the extracellular space.
6. Potassium and magnesium are the most common electrolytes in the intracellular space.
7. Oncotic pressure arises from the presence of plasma proteins and other large high molecular weight particles within the vascular space.
8. d. Cardiac output and blood pressure

Chapter 2

1. Hypovolemia is a deficit in circulating fluid volume.
2. Any three of the following: skin tent, eye position, mucous membrane moisture, or mentation.
3. A decrease in circulating volume leads to decreased stroke volume. Because cardiac output is the product of stroke volume and heart rate, a decrease in stroke volume

Fluid Therapy for Veterinary Technicians and Nurses, First Edition. Charlotte Donohoe.
© 2012 Charlotte Donohoe. Published 2012 by John Wiley & Sons, Inc.

leads to a decrease in cardiac output. As such, hypovolemia leads to decreased cardiac output.

4. The goal of the physiologic changes seen with hypovolemia is to maintain tissue perfusion and preserve organ function.

5. Palpation of one femoral pulse and not the other can fail to identify arterial thrombosis affecting the quality of one femoral pulse and not the other.

6. Dorsal pedal pulses are thought to disappear when the patient's mean arterial pressure is less than or equal to 60 mm Hg. One can assume that if there is no palpable dorsal pedal pulse, the patient is hypotensive and possibly hypovolemic.

7. a. Dehydration

   b. Protein loss

   c. Splenic contraction

8. a. High

   b. The kidneys conserve water in times of dehydration. If the same solutes are excreted in a smaller volume of urine, the USG is higher due to the increased solute concentration.

Chapter 3

1. Animals that suffer from conditions involving vomiting, diarrhea, abdominal distension or decreased motility are not candidates for enteral fluid therapy.

2. The tube must be measured to ensure that the proximal end reaches beyond the nasopharynx and into the esophagus.

3. The tube is measured from the tip of the nose to the seventh intercostal space.

4. An animal can safely receive 10 mL/kg of fluids at each SC injection site.

5. Patients with marked hypotension, marked dehydration, or hypothermia are not candidates for SC fluids. Circulation to the periphery and skin is diminished during these conditions, which will inhibit distribution of fluids delivered by this route.

6. Any two of the following: The IO compartment doesn't collapse; fluids are quickly redistributed; can deliver high volume and can deliver at fast rate; can deliver same fluids as IV route.

7. IO catheters can be difficult to place due to challenges associated with identifying proper landmarks. Osteomyelitis is also a potential complication with IO catheter placement.

8. Cephalic vein, lateral saphenous vein, medial saphenous vein, jugular vein

9. Polyurethane

Chapter 4

1. By positioning the line in this manner, the technician avoids air traveling into the line and subsequently into the patient.

2. 10 gtt/s and 60 gtt/s

3. An inline filter must be used when the patient is receiving blood products.

4. Smaller volume syringes are safer because back pressure is recognized more quickly in the smaller volume syringe and a line occlusion alarm will sound sooner than with a larger volume syringe.

5. Any of the following are acceptable answers:
   a. Preset volumes avoid infusion of excess volume in an emergency setting.
   b. Burettes can be used for constant rates of infusion.
   c. Burettes can facilitate quick changes of drug concentrations.
   d. Burettes can be used for slow infusion of medications.
   e. Burettes are far less expensive than syringe pumps or syringe drivers.

Chapter 5

1. The technician should add 10.5 mL of KCl to the remaining 700 mL of IV fluid in the bag.
2. The dog will receive 1.5 mL/h of fentanyl.
3. A total of 12 mL of fentanyl is added to the bag to provide 1.5 mL/h of fentanyl for 8 hours of fluid left in the bag.
4. Adding 10 mL of 50% dextrose to the IV fluids in the burette will provide a solution of 5% dextrose. (Note: Some clinics prefer to remove 10 mL of IV fluids so that the total volume is 100 mL and the 5% dextrose solution is slightly more accurate.)
5. A total of 8.3 mL of metoclopramide should be added to a 1-L bag of fluids to provide this patient with 2 mg/kg per day of metoclopramide at a fluid rate of 50 mL/h.

Chapter 6

1. Patients that have recently undergone rectal surgery are not suitable candidates for continuous temperature measurement via rectal probe. In addition, animals with severe coagulopathies should not be monitored using these probes. Patients that are extremely aggressive might also be unsuitable candidates for this type of monitoring.
2. Pyrexia describes an elevated body temperature that arises when the body attempts to defend itself (e.g., against infection). In this condition, the body's regulation of temperature is disrupted and reset. Hyperthermia refers to any condition in which body temperature is elevated above normal.
3. *Tachycardia* is the term used to describe a heart rate elevated beyond what is normally expected for a particular animal.
4. Bradycardia describes a heart rate that is slower than what is normally acceptable for a given patient.
5. Serial body weight measurement, measurement of urine output, and calculation of fluids IN compared to fluids OUT are all acceptable ways of estimating fluid loss or gain in a hospitalized patient.
6. A total of 500 g of body weight is comparable with a volume of approximately 500 mL of fluid.
7. b. Hypovolemia
8. b. An increase in circulating volume
9. 1–2 mL/kg

Chapter 7

1. d. Inflammation of a blood vessel
2. blood clot
3. c. Coagulopathic patients
4. Any three of the following: increased respiratory rate; restlessness; increased heart rate; increased urine output; chemosis, edema; nasal discharge; vomiting and diarrhea.
5. Peripheral edema

Chapter 8

1. Any three of the following: small low molecular weight particles; move freely throughout body compartments; enter interstitial compartment quickly; do not contribute to oncotic pressure; do contribute to osmotic pressure.
2. Maintenance crystalloids contain *less* sodium than replacement crystalloids.
3. a. higher than
4. Hypertonic saline increases osmotic pressure and draws fluid into the intravascular space. This is helpful in patients whose intravascular space is lacking in volume.
5. The large molecular weight particles remain in the intravascular space creating an increase in oncotic pressure. The increased oncotic pressure helps draw fluid from other body water compartments into the vascular space.
6. HTS and colloids draw fluid into the vascular space. If capillaries are leaky or damaged and HTS or colloids leave the vascular space, they will draw fluids into the compartment into which they have passed. This can lead to interstitial edema, pulmonary edema, and other complications detrimental to patient health.

Chapter 9

1. The technician can evaluate mucous membrane color, capillary refill time, heart rate, and pulse quality.
2. Skin tent; eye position; mucous membrane moisture
3. Replacement fluids
4. Plasma-Lyte A, Normosol R, and lactated Ringer solution would all be appropriate in this situation.
5. Restore intravascular volume; restore perfusion; treat hypovolemia

Chapter 10

1. A means to deliver nutrition via the intravenous route to patients that are unable to receive it by the oral route or via their gastrointestinal tract.
2. TPN delivers 100% of the patient's nutritional requirements; PPN delivers 50% of the patient's nutritional requirements.

3. There are many different reasons to consider that a patient might benefit from PN. The most common guidelines include the following:
   a. The patient has been anorexic for 3 days
   b. The patient is expected to be anorexic for at least 3 days
   c. The patient's illness is such that the animal is expected to lose muscle mass during hospitalization
   d. The patient has undergone gastrointestinal surgery or is unable to receive enteral nutrition.
4. Any of the following complications can arise: catheter occlusion, kinking of administration sets, compromise of sterility (patient soiling of lines), infection, hyperglycemia, hypoglycemia, or refeeding syndrome (rare).
5. A condition that arises when an animal that has been without nutrition for a prolonged period of time finally receives some form of feeding. The animal's body carries out a variety of physiologic processes that ultimately can result in some important electrolyte disturbances. The disturbances most commonly seen in refeeding syndrome are hypophosphatemia, hypokalemia, and hypomagnesemia.

Chapter 11

1. They should be between 1 and 7 years of age and weigh at least 22 kg.
2. Cats should be between 1 and 7 years of age and weigh at least 4.5 kg.
3. DEA 1.1 and DEA 1.2 are the most important antigens to identify when blood typing donors and recipients.
4. Cats have either blood type A, B, or AB. The most common blood type in cats is type A.
5. The bags contain citrate phosphate dextrose adenine (CPDA).
6. CPDA is an anticoagulant and preservative that maintains the integrity of the cells while prolonging their shelf life.
7. Packed red blood cells would be the ideal choice for this patient because what the animal requires most is the red blood cells.
8. The patient's temperature, pulse, and respiration are measured both before and after the test dose. Increases in any of these vital signs after the test dose warrant close monitoring and may indicate that the patient is having a reaction to the blood product being administered.
9. Autotransfusion refers to the intravenous delivery of whole blood that has been collected from a body cavity of the same patient. The blood is collected into an anticoagulant-loaded closed collection system and can be given back to the patient. The blood is administered through an inline filter to ensure no clots are delivered intravenously.

Index

Page numbers in *italics* represent figures; those in **bold**, tables.

Fluid Therapy for Veterinary Technicians and Nurses, First Edition. Charlotte Donohoe.
© 2012 Charlotte Donohoe. Published 2012 by John Wiley & Sons, Inc.